Breakfast and Brunch the Mediterranean Way

Kickstart Your Day With A Taste of the Mediterranean Sea

By
Delia Bell

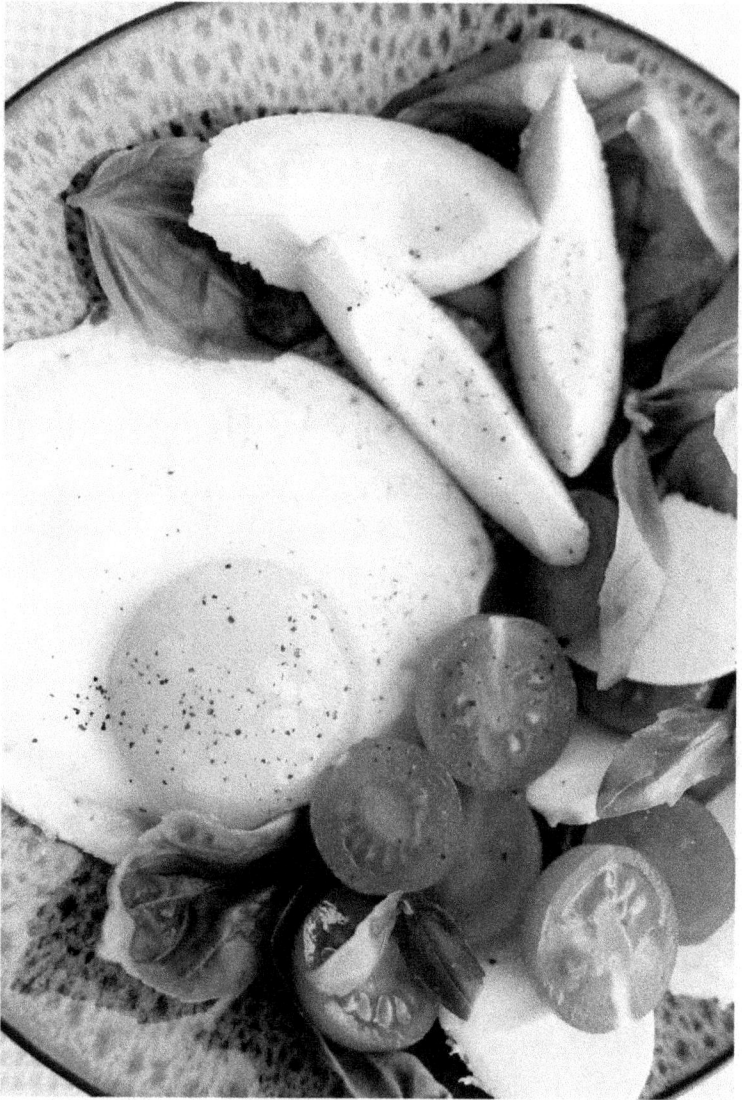

the publisher or the original author of this work can be in any fashion deemed liable for any hardship or damages that may befall them after undertaking information described herein.

Additionally, the information in the following pages is intended only for informational purposes and should thus be thought of as universal. As befitting its nature, it is presented without assurance regarding its prolonged validity or interim quality. Trademarks that are mentioned are done without written consent and can in no way be considered an endorsement from the trademark holder.

Table of Contents

INTRODUCTION

What is the Mediterranean Diet?

The Mediterranean diet is based on the diets of traditional eating habits from the 1960s of people from countries that surround the Mediterranean Sea, such as Greece, Italy, and Spain, and it encourages the consumption of fresh, seasonal, and local foods. The Mediterranean diet has become popular because individuals show low rates of heart disease, chronic disease, and obesity. The Mediterranean diet profile focuses on whole grains, good fats (fish, olive oil, nuts etc.), vegetables, fruits, fish, and very low consumption of any non-fish meat. Along with food, the Mediterranean diet emphasizes the need to spend time eating with family and physical activity. The Mediterranean diet is not a single prescribed diet, but rather a general food-based eating pattern, which is marked by local and cultural differences throughout the Mediterranean region.

The diet is generally characterized by a high intake of plant-based foods (e.g. fresh fruit and vegetables, nuts, and cereals) and olive oil, a moderate intake of fish and poultry, and low intakes of dairy products (mostly yoghurt and cheese), red and processed meats, and sweets. Wine is typically consumed in moderation and, normally, with a meal. A strong focus is placed on social and cultural aspects, such as communal mealtimes, resting after eating, and regular physical activity. Nowadays, however, the diet is no longer followed as widely as it was 30-50 years ago, as the diets of people living in these regions are becoming more 'Westernized' and higher in energy dense foods.

Benefits

The Mediterranean diet is not a weight loss, but increasing fiber intake and cutting out red meat, animal fats, and processed food may lead to weight loss. People who follow the diet may also have a lower risk of various diseases.

Heart health

In the 1950s,an American scientist, found that people living in the poorer areas of southern Italy had a lower risk of heart disease and death than those in wealthier parts of New York. Dr. Keys attributed this to diet. Since then, many studies have indicated that following a Mediterranean diet can help the body maintain healthy cholesterol levels and reduce the risk of high blood pressure and cardiovascular disease. The overall pattern of the Mediterranean diet is similar to their own dietary recommendations. A high proportion of calories on the diet come from fat, which can increase the risk of obesity.

However, they also note that this fat is mainly unsaturated, which makes it a more healthful option than that from the typical American diet.

Protection from disease
The Mediterranean diet focuses on plant-based foods, and these are good sources of antioxidants.

The Mediterranean diet might offer protection from various cancers, and especially colorectal cancer. The reduction in risk may stem from the high intake of fruits, vegetables, and whole grains. By sticking to Mediterranean meals, people's levels of blood glucose and fats had decreased. During this time, there was also a lower incidence of stroke.

Diabetes
The Mediterranean diet may help prevent type 2 diabetes and improve markers of diabetes in people who already have the condition. Various other studies have concluded that following the Mediterranean diet can reduce the risk of type 2 diabetes and cardiovascular disease, which often occur together.

Food to eat
There is no single definition of the Mediterranean diet, but one group of scientists used the following as their 2015

basis of research.

Vegetables: Include 3 to 9 servings a day.

Fresh fruit: Up to 2 servings a day.

Cereals: Mostly whole grain from 1 to 13 servings a day.

Oil: Up to 8 servings of extra virgin (cold pressed) olive oil a day.

Fat — mostly unsaturated — made up 37% of the total calories. Unsaturated fat comes from plant sources, such as olives and avocado. The Mediterranean diet also provided 33 grams (g) of fiber a day. The baseline diet for this study provided around 2,200 calories a day. Typical ingredients. Here are some examples of ingredients that people often include in the Mediterranean diet.

Vegetables: Tomatoes, peppers, onions, eggplant, zucchini, cucumber, leafy green vegetables, plus others.

Fruits: Melon, apples, apricots, peaches, oranges, and lemons, and so on.

Legumes: Beans, lentils, and chickpeas.

Nuts and seeds: Almonds, walnuts, sunflower seeds, and cashews.

Unsaturated fat: Olive oil, sunflower oil, olives, and avocados.

Dairy products: Cheese and yogurt are the main dairy

foods.

Cereals: These are mostly whole grain and include wheat and rice with bread accompanying many meals.

Fish: Sardines and other oily fish, as well as oysters and other shellfish. Poultry: Chicken or turkey.

Eggs: Chicken, quail, and duck eggs.

Drinks: A person can drink red wine in moderation.

The Mediterranean diet does not include strong liquor or carbonated and sweetened drinks. According to one definition, the diet limits red meat and sweets to less than 2 servings per week.

Food to avoid
Here's a list of foods you should generally limit while eating Mediterranean-style meals. Heavily processed foods. Let's be real: Many, many foods are processed to some degree. A can of beans has been processed, in the sense that the beans have been cooked before being canned. Olive oil has been processed, because olives have been turned into oil. But when we talk about limiting processed foods, this really means avoiding things like frozen meals with tons of sodium. You should also limit soda, desserts and candy. As the adage goes, if the ingredient list includes items that

your great-grandparents wouldn't recognize as food, it's probably processed. If you're buying a packaged food that's as close to its whole-food form as possible — such as frozen fruit or veggies with nothing added — you're good to go.

Processed red meat

On the Mediterranean diet, you should minimize your intake of red meat, such as steak. What about processed red meat, such as hot dogs and bacon? You should avoid these foods or limit them as much as possible. A study published in BMJ found that regularly eating red meat, especially processed varieties, was associated with a higher risk of death. Butter. Here's another food that should be limited on the Mediterranean diet. Use olive oil instead, which has many heart health benefits and contains less saturated fat than butter. According to the USDA National Nutrient Database, butter has 7 grams of saturated fat per tablespoon, while olive oil has about 2 grams.

Refined grains

The Mediterranean diet is centered around whole grains, such as farro, millet, couscous and brown rice. With this eating style, you'll generally want to limit your intake of refined grains such as white pasta and white bread.

Alcohol

When you're following the Mediterranean diet, red wine should be your chosen alcoholic drink. This is because red wine offers health benefits, particularly for the heart. But it's important to limit intake of any type of alcohol to up to one drink per day for women, as well as men older than 65, and up to two drinks daily for men age 65 and younger. The amount that counts as a drink is 5 ounces of wine, 12 ounces of beer or 1.5 ounces of 80-proof liquor.

Zucchini And Quinoa Pan

Servings: 4
Cooking Time: 20 Minutes

Ingredients:
- 1 tablespoon olive oil
- 2 garlic cloves, minced
- 1 cup quinoa
- 1 zucchini, roughly cubed
- 2 tablespoons basil, chopped
- ¼ cup green olives, pitted and chopped
- 1 tomato, cubed
- ½ cup feta cheese, crumbled
- 2 cups water
- 1 cup canned garbanzo beans, drained and rinsed
- A pinch of salt and black pepper

Directions:
1. Heat up a pan with the oil over medium-high heat, add the garlic and quinoa and brown for 3 minutes.
2. Add the water, zucchinis, salt and pepper, toss, bring to a simmer and cook for 15 minutes.
3. Add the rest of the ingredients, toss, divide everything between plates and serve for breakfast.

Nutrition Info: calories 310, fat 11, fiber 6, carbs 42, protein 11

Peas Omelet

Servings: 6

Cooking Time: 20 Minutes

Ingredients:

- 4 oz green peas
- ¼ cup corn kernels
- 6 eggs, beaten
- ¼ cup heavy cream
- ½ teaspoon of sea salt
- 1 red bell pepper, chopped
- 1 teaspoon butter
- ½ teaspoon paprika

Directions:

1. Toss butter in the skillet and melt it.

2. Add green peas, bell pepper, and corn kernels. Start to roast the vegetables over the medium heat.

3. Meanwhile, in the mixing bowl whisk together eggs, heavy cream, sea salt, and paprika.

4. Pour the mixture over the roasted vegetables and stir well immediately.

5. Close the lid and cook omelet over the medium-low heat for 15 minutes or until it is solid.

6. Transfer the cooked omelet in the big plate and cut into the servings.

Nutrition Info:Per Serving:calories 113, fat 7.1, fiber 1.5, carbs 6, protein 7.1 3. Low Carb

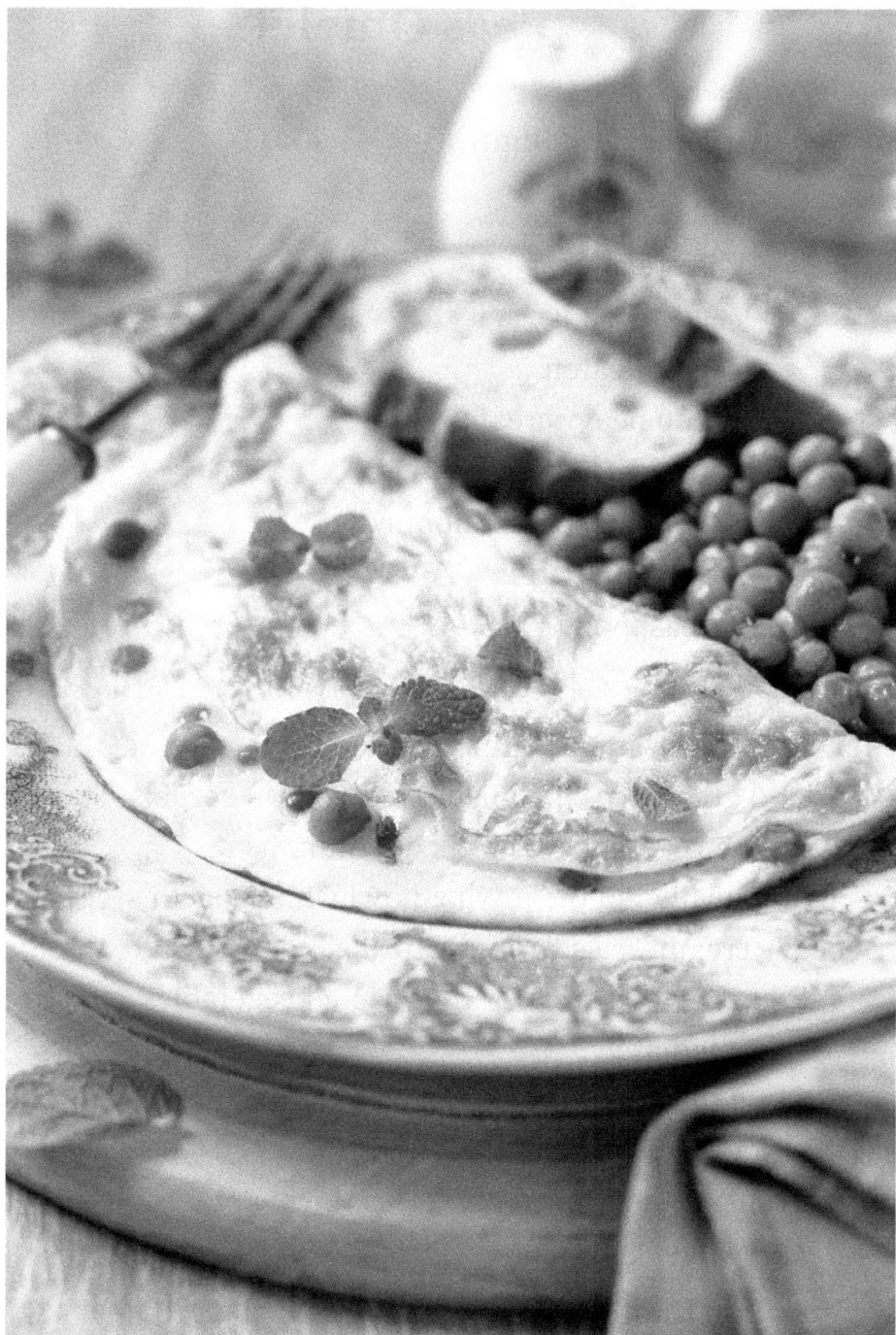

Green Smoothie

Servings: 2
Cooking Time: 15 Mins

Ingredients:
- 1/3 cup romaine lettuce
- 1/3 tablespoon fresh ginger, peeled and chopped
- 1½ cups filtered water
- 1/8 cup fresh pineapple, chopped
- ¾ tablespoon fresh parsley
- 1/3 cup raw cucumber, peeled and sliced
- ¼ Hass avocado
- ¼ cup kiwi fruit, peeled and chopped
- 1/3 tablespoon Swerve

Directions:
1. Put all the ingredients in a blender and blend until smooth.
2. Pour into 2 serving glasses and serve chilled.

Nutrition Info: Calories: 108 Carbs: 7.8g Fats: 8.9g Proteins: 1.6g Sodium: 4mg Sugar: 2.2g

Fig With Ricotta Oatmeal

Servings: 1

Cooking Time: 5 Minutes

Ingredients:

- 2 teaspoons honey
- 2 tablespoons ricotta cheese, part-skim
- 2 tablespoons dried figs, chopped
- 1/2 cup old-fashioned rolled oats
- 1 tablespoon almonds, toasted, sliced
- 1 cup water
- Pinch of salt

Directions:

1. Pour the water in a small saucepan and add the salt; bring to a boil.

2. Stir in the oats and reduce heat to medium. Cook the oats for about 5 minutes, occasionally stirring, until most of the water is absorbed.

3. Remove the pan from the heat, cover, and let stand for 2-3 minutes.

4. Serve topped with the figs, almonds, ricotta, and drizzle of honey.

Nutrition Info:Per Serving:315 Cal, 8 g total fat (2 g sat. fat, 4 g mono), 10 mg chol., 194 mg sodium, 359 mg pot., 53 g carb.,7 g fiber, 10 g protein.

Raspberry Pudding

Servings: 2

Cooking Time: 30 Minutes

Ingredients:

- ½ cup raspberries
- 2 teaspoons maple syrup
- 1 ½ cup Plain yogurt
- ¼ teaspoon ground cardamom
- 1/3 cup Chia seeds, dried

Directions:

1. Mix together plain yogurt with maple syrup and ground cardamom.
2. Add Chia seeds. Stir it gently.
3. Put the yogurt in the serving glasses and top with the raspberries.
4. Refrigerate the breakfast for at least 30 minutes or overnight.

Nutrition Info:Per Serving:calories 303, fat 11.2, fiber 11.8, carbs 33.2, protein 15.5

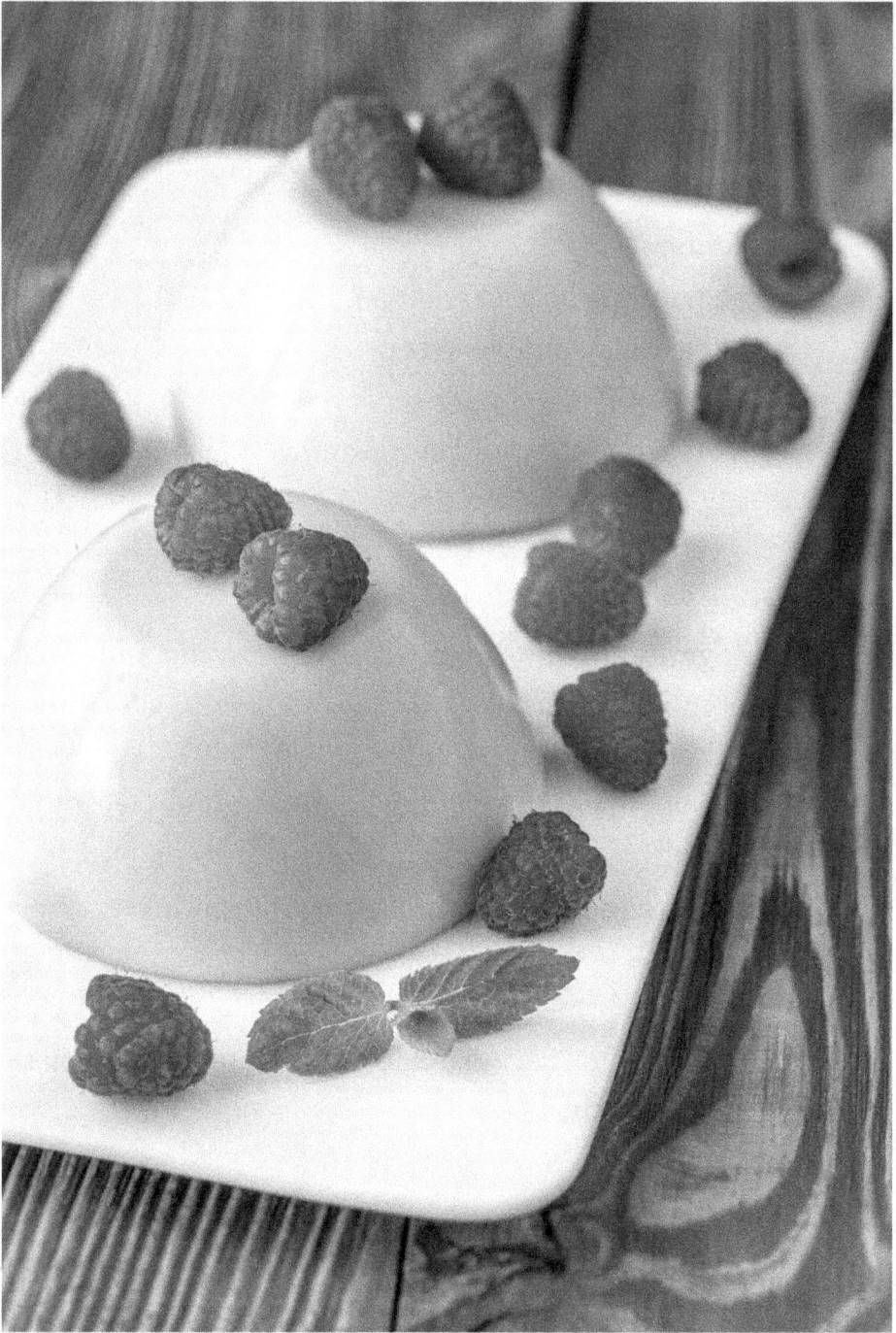

Walnuts Yogurt Mix

Servings: 6
Cooking Time: 0 Minutes

Ingredients:
- 2 and ½ cups Greek yogurt
- 1 and ½ cups walnuts, chopped
- 1 teaspoon vanilla extract
- ¾ cup honey
- 2 teaspoons cinnamon powder

Directions:
1. In a bowl, combine the yogurt with the walnuts and the rest of the ingredients, toss, divide into smaller bowls and keep in the fridge for 10 minutes before serving for breakfast.

Nutrition Info: calories 388, fat 24.6, fiber 2.9, carbs 39.1, protein 10.2

Egg-feta Scramble

Servings: 4
Cooking Time: 15 Minutes

Ingredients:
- 6 eggs
- 3/4 cup crumbled feta cheese
- 2 tablespoons green onions, minced
- 2 tablespoons red peppers, roasted, diced
- 1/4 teaspoon kosher salt
- 1/4 teaspoon garlic powder
- 1/4 cup Greek yogurt
- 1/2 teaspoon dry oregano
- 1/2 teaspoon dry basil
- 1 teaspoon olive oil
- A few cracks freshly ground black pepper
- Warm whole-wheat tortillas, optional

Directions:
1. Preheat a skillet over medium heat.
2. In a bowl, whisk the eggs, the sour cream, basil, oregano, garlic powder, salt, and pepper. Gently add the feta.
3. When the skillet is hot, add the olive oil and then the egg mixture; allow the egg mix to set then scrape the bottom of the pan to let the uncooked egg to cook. Stir in the red peppers and the green onions. Continue cooking until the

eggs mixture is cooked to your preferred doneness. Serve immediately.

4. If desired, sprinkle with extra feta and then wrap the scrambled eggs in tortillas.

Nutrition Info:Per Serving:260 Cal, 16 g total fat (8 g sat. fat), 350 mg chol., 750 mg sodium, 190 mg pot., 12 g carb.,>1 g fiber, 2 g sugar, 16 g protein.

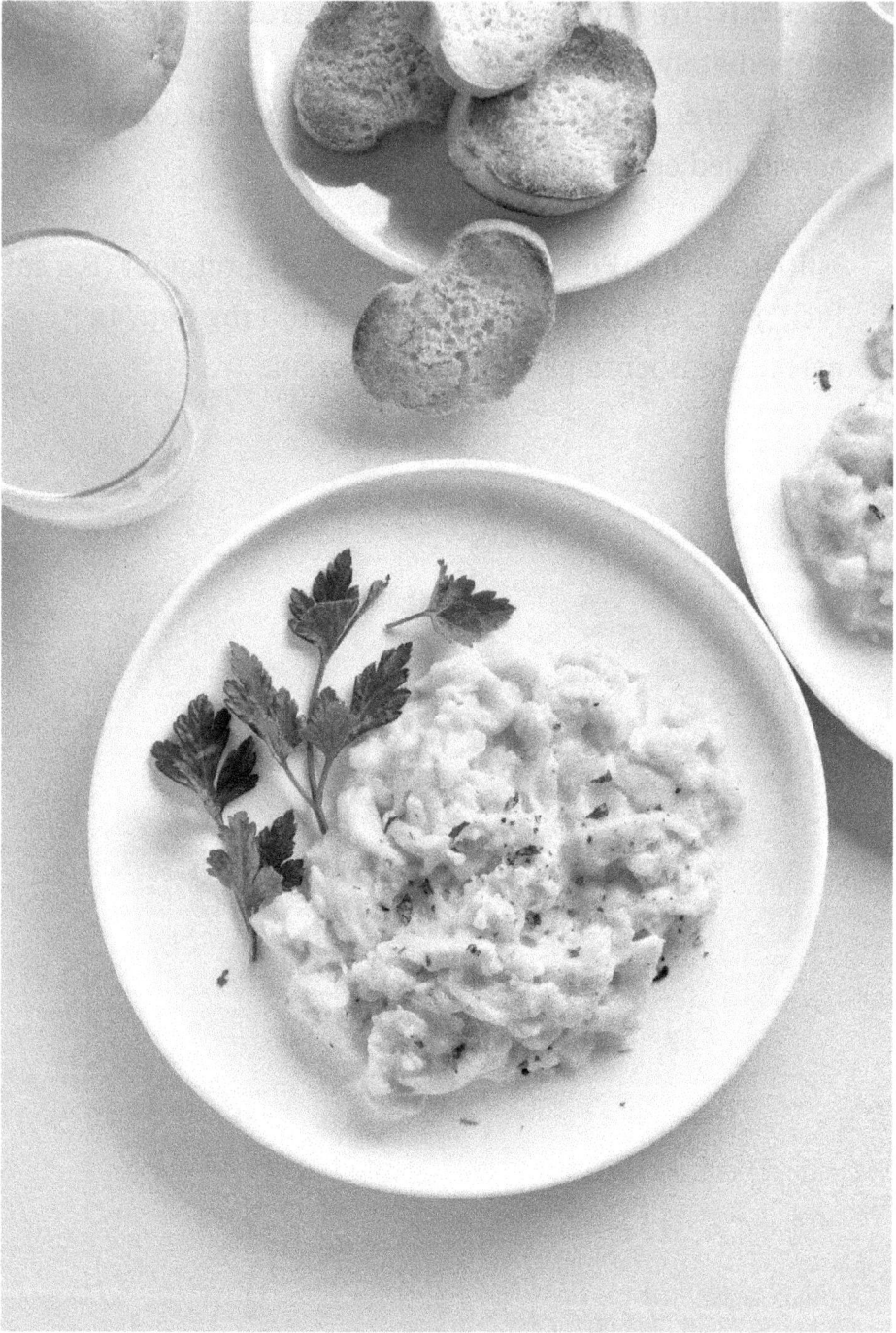

Spiced Chickpeas Bowls

Servings: 4
Cooking Time: 30 Minutes

Ingredients:

- 15 ounces canned chickpeas, drained and rinsed
- ¼ teaspoon cardamom, ground
- ½ teaspoon cinnamon powder
- 1 and ½ teaspoons turmeric powder
- 1 teaspoon coriander, ground
- 1 tablespoon olive oil
- A pinch of salt and black pepper
- ¾ cup Greek yogurt
- ½ cup green olives, pitted and halved
- ½ cup cherry tomatoes, halved
- 1 cucumber, sliced

Directions:
1. Spread the chickpeas on a lined baking sheet, add the cardamom, cinnamon, turmeric, coriander, the oil, salt and pepper, toss and bake at 375 degrees F for 30 minutes.
2. In a bowl, combine the roasted chickpeas with the rest of the ingredients, toss and serve for breakfast.

Nutrition Info: calories 519, fat 34.5, fiber 13.3, carbs 49.8, protein 12

Orzo And Veggie Bowls

Servings: 4

Cooking Time: 0 Minutes

Ingredients:

- 2 and ½ cups whole-wheat orzo, cooked
- 14 ounces canned cannellini beans, drained and rinsed
- 1 yellow bell pepper, cubed
- 1 green bell pepper, cubed
- A pinch of salt and black pepper
- 3 tomatoes, cubed
- 1 red onion, chopped
- 1 cup mint, chopped
- 2 cups feta cheese, crumbled
- 2 tablespoons olive oil
- ¼ cup lemon juice
- 1 tablespoon lemon zest, grated
- 1 cucumber, cubed
- 1 and ¼ cup kalamata olives, pitted and sliced
- 3 garlic cloves, minced

Directions:

1. In a salad bowl, combine the orzo with the beans, bell peppers and the rest of the ingredients, toss, divide the mix between plates and serve for breakfast.

Nutrition Info: calories 411, fat 17, fiber 13, carbs 51, protein 14

Vanilla Oats

Servings: 4
Cooking Time: 10 Minutes

Ingredients:
- ½ cup rolled oats
- 1 cup milk
- 1 teaspoon vanilla extract
- 1 teaspoon ground cinnamon
- 2 teaspoon honey
- 2 tablespoons Plain yogurt
- 1 teaspoon butter

Directions:
1. Pour milk in the saucepan and bring it to boil.
2. Add rolled oats and stir well.
3. Close the lid and simmer the oats for 5 minutes over the medium heat. The cooked oats will absorb all milk.
4. Then add butter and stir the oats well.
5. In the separated bowl, whisk together Plain yogurt with honey, cinnamon, and vanilla extract.
6. Transfer the cooked oats in the serving bowls.
7. Top the oats with the yogurt mixture in the shape of the wheel.

Nutrition Info:Per Serving:calories 243, fat 20.2, fiber 1, carbs 2.8, protein 13.3

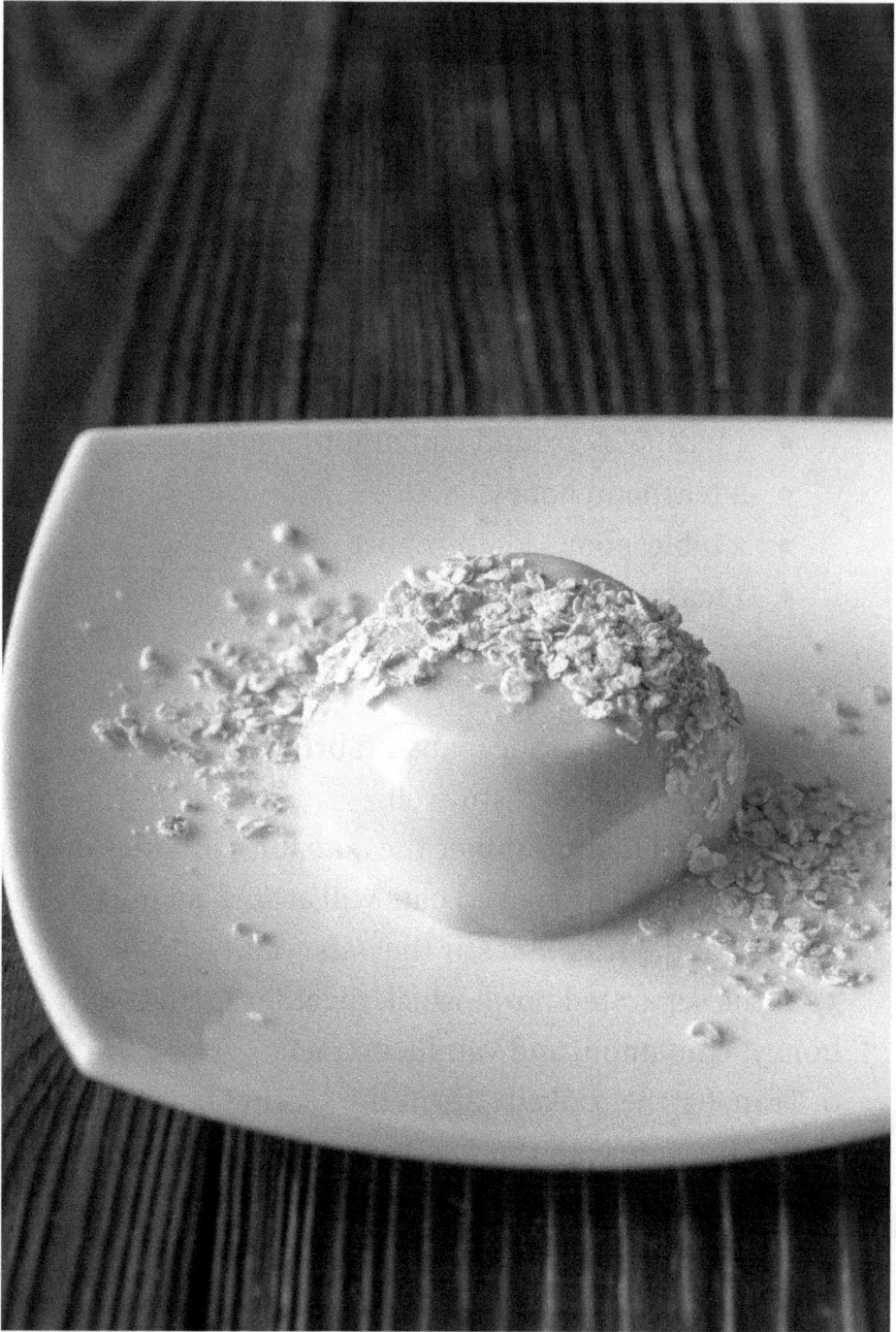

Casserole

Servings: 3
Cooking Time: 25 Minutes

Ingredients:
- ½ cup mushrooms, chopped
- ½ yellow onion, diced
- 4 eggs, beaten
- 1 tablespoon coconut flakes
- ½ teaspoon chili pepper
- 1 oz Cheddar cheese, shredded
- 1 teaspoon canola oil

Directions:
1. Pour canola oil in the skillet and preheat well.
2. Add mushrooms and onion and roast for 5-8 minutes or until the vegetables are light brown.
3. Transfer the cooked vegetables in the casserole mold.
4. Add coconut flakes, chili pepper, and Cheddar cheese.
5. Then add eggs and stir well.
6. Bake the casserole for 15 minutes at 360F.

Nutrition Info: Calories 152, fat 11.1, fiber 0.7, carbs 3, protein 10.4

Bacon Veggies Combo

Servings: 2

Cooking Time: 35 Minutes

Ingredients:

- ½ green bell pepper, seeded and chopped
- 2 bacon slices
- ¼ cup Parmesan Cheese
- ½ tablespoon mayonnaise
- 1 scallion, chopped

Directions:

1. Preheat the oven to 375 degrees F and grease a baking dish.
2. Place bacon slices on the baking dish and top with mayonnaise, bell peppers, scallions and Parmesan Cheese.
3. Transfer in the oven and bake for about 25 minutes.
4. Dish out to serve immediately or refrigerate for about 2 days wrapped in a plastic sheet for meal prepping.

Nutrition Info: Calories: 197 Fat: 13.8g Carbohydrates: 4.7g Protein: 14.3g Sugar: 1.9g Sodium: 662mg

Brown Rice Salad

Servings: 4

Cooking Time: 0 Minutes

Ingredients:

- 9 ounces brown rice, cooked
- 7 cups baby arugula
- 15 ounces canned garbanzo beans, drained and rinsed
- 4 ounces feta cheese, crumbled
- ¾ cup basil, chopped
- A pinch of salt and black pepper
- 2 tablespoons lemon juice
- ¼ teaspoon lemon zest, grated
- ¼ cup olive oil

Directions:

1. In a salad bowl, combine the brown rice with the arugula, the beans and the rest of the ingredients, toss and serve cold for breakfast.

Nutrition Info: calories 473, fat 22, fiber 7, carbs 53, protein 13

Olive And Milk Bread

Servings: 6
Cooking Time: 50 Minutes

Ingredients:
- 1 cup black olives, pitted, chopped
- 1 tablespoon olive oil
- ½ teaspoon fresh yeast
- ½ cup milk, preheated
- ½ teaspoon salt
- 1 teaspoon baking powder
- 2 cup wheat flour, whole grain
- 2 eggs, beaten
- 1 teaspoon butter, melted
- 1 teaspoon sugar

Directions:
1. In the big bowl combine together fresh yeast, sugar, and milk. Stir it until yeast is dissolved.
2. Then add salt, baking powder, butter, and eggs. Stir the dough mixture until homogenous and add 1 cup of wheat flour. Mix it up until smooth.
3. Add olives and remaining flour. Knead the non-sticky dough.
4. Transfer the dough into the non-sticky dough mold.
5. Bake the bread for 50 minutes at 350 F.

6. Check if the bread is cooked with the help of the toothpick. If it is dry, the bread is cooked.

7. Remove the bread from the oven and let it chill for 10-15 minutes.

8. Remove it from the loaf mold and slice.

Nutrition Info:Per Serving:calories 238, fat 7.7, fiber 1.9, carbs 35.5, protein 7.2

Breakfast Tostadas

Servings: 6
Cooking Time: 6 Minutes

Ingredients:
- ½ white onion, diced
- 1 tomato, chopped
- 1 cucumber, chopped
- 1 tablespoon fresh cilantro, chopped
- ½ jalapeno pepper, chopped
- 1 tablespoon lime juice
- 6 corn tortillas
- 1 tablespoon canola oil
- 2 oz Cheddar cheese, shredded
- ½ cup white beans, canned, drained
- 6 eggs
- ½ teaspoon butter
- ½ teaspoon Sea salt

Directions:
1. Make Pico de Galo: in the salad bowl combine together diced white onion, tomato, cucumber, fresh cilantro, and jalapeno pepper.
2. Then add lime juice and a ½ tablespoon of canola oil. Mix up the mixture well. Pico de Galo is cooked.
3. After this, preheat the oven to 390F.
4. Line the tray with baking paper.

5. Arrange the corn tortillas on the baking paper and brush with remaining canola oil from both sides.

6. Bake the tortillas for 10 minutes or until they start to be crunchy.

7. Chill the cooked crunchy tortillas well.

8. Meanwhile, toss the butter in the skillet.

9. Crack the eggs in the melted butter and sprinkle them with sea salt.

10. Fry the eggs until the egg whites become white (cooked). Approximately for 3-5 minutes over the medium heat.

11. After this, mash the beans until you get puree texture.

12. Spread the bean puree on the corn tortillas.

13. Add fried eggs.

14. Then top the eggs with Pico de Galo and shredded Cheddar cheese.

Nutrition Info: Calories 246, fat 11.1, fiber 4.7, carbs 24.5, protein 13.7

Chicken Souvlaki

Servings: 4
Cooking Time: 2 Minutes

Ingredients:
- 4 pieces (6-inch) pitas, cut into halves
- 2 cups roasted chicken breast skinless, boneless, and sliced
- 1/4 cup red onion, thinly sliced
- 1/2 teaspoon dried oregano
- 1/2 cup Greek yogurt, plain
- 1/2 cup plum tomato, chopped
- 1/2 cup cucumber, peeled, chopped
- 1/2 cup (2 ounces) feta cheese, crumbled
- 1 tablespoon olive oil, extra-virgin, divided
- 1 tablespoon fresh dill, chopped
- 1 cup iceberg lettuce, shredded
- 1 1/4 teaspoons minced garlic, bottled, divided

Directions:
1. In a small mixing bowl, combine the yogurt, cheese, 1 teaspoon of the olive oil, and 1/4 teaspoon of the garlic until well mixed.
2. In a large skillet, heat the remaining olive oil over medium-high heat. Add the remaining 1 teaspoon garlic and the oregano; sauté for 20 seconds.

3. Add the chicken; cook for about 2 minutes or until the chicken is heated through.

4. Put 1/4 cup chicken into each pita halves. Top with 2 tablespoons yogurt mix, 2 tablespoons lettuce,1 tablespoon tomato, and 1 tablespoon cucumber. Divide the onion between the pita halves.

Nutrition Info:Per Serving:414 Cal, 13.7 g total fat (6.4 g sat. fat, 1.4 g poly. Fat, 4.7 g mono), 81 mg chol., 595 mg sodium, 38 g carb.,2 g fiber, 32.3 g protein.

Tahini Pine Nuts Toast

Servings: 2

Cooking Time: 0 Minutes

Ingredients:

- 2 whole wheat bread slices, toasted
- 1 teaspoon water
- 1 tablespoon tahini paste
- 2 teaspoons feta cheese, crumbled
- Juice of ½ lemon
- 2 teaspoons pine nuts
- A pinch of black pepper

Directions:

1. In a bowl, mix the tahini with the water and the lemon juice, whisk really well and spread over the toasted bread slices.

2. Top each serving with the remaining ingredients and serve for breakfast.

Nutrition Info: calories 142, fat 7.6, fiber 2.7, carbs 13.7, protein 5.8

Eggs And Veggies

Servings: 4
Cooking Time: 15 Minutes

Ingredients:
- 2 tomatoes, chopped
- 2 eggs, beaten
- 1 bell pepper, chopped
- 1 teaspoon tomato paste
- ¼ cup of water
- 1 teaspoon butter
- ½ white onion, diced
- ½ teaspoon chili flakes
- 1/3 teaspoon sea salt

Directions:
1. Put butter in the pan and melt it.
2. Add bell pepper and cook it for 3 minutes over the medium heat. Stir it
from time to time.
3. After this, add diced onion and cook it for 2 minutes more.
4. Stir the vegetables and add tomatoes.
5. Cook them for 5 minutes over the medium-low heat.
6. Then add water and tomato paste. Stir well.
7. Add beaten eggs, chili flakes, and sea salt.

8. Stir well and cook menemen for 4 minutes over the medium-low heat.

9. The cooked meal should be half runny.

Nutrition Info:Per Serving:calories 67, fat 3.4, fiber 1.5, carbs 6.4, protein 3.8

Chili Scramble

Servings: 4
Cooking Time: 15 Minutes

Ingredients:
- 3 tomatoes
- 4 eggs
- ¼ teaspoon of sea salt
- ½ chili pepper, chopped
- 1 tablespoon butter
- 1 cup water, for cooking

Directions:
1. Pour water in the saucepan and bring it to boil.
2. Then remove water from the heat and add tomatoes.
3. Let the tomatoes stay in the hot water for 2-3 minutes.
4. After this, remove the tomatoes from water and peel them.
5. Place butter in the pan and melt it.
6. Add chopped chili pepper and fry it for 3 minutes over the medium heat.
7. Then chop the peeled tomatoes and add into the chili peppers.
8. Cook the vegetables for 5 minutes over the medium heat. Stir them from time to time.
9. After this, add sea salt and crack the eggs.

10. Stir (scramble) the eggs well with the help of the fork and cook them for 3 minutes over the medium heat.

Nutrition Info:Per Serving:calories 105, fat 7.4, fiber 1.1, carbs 4, protein 6.4

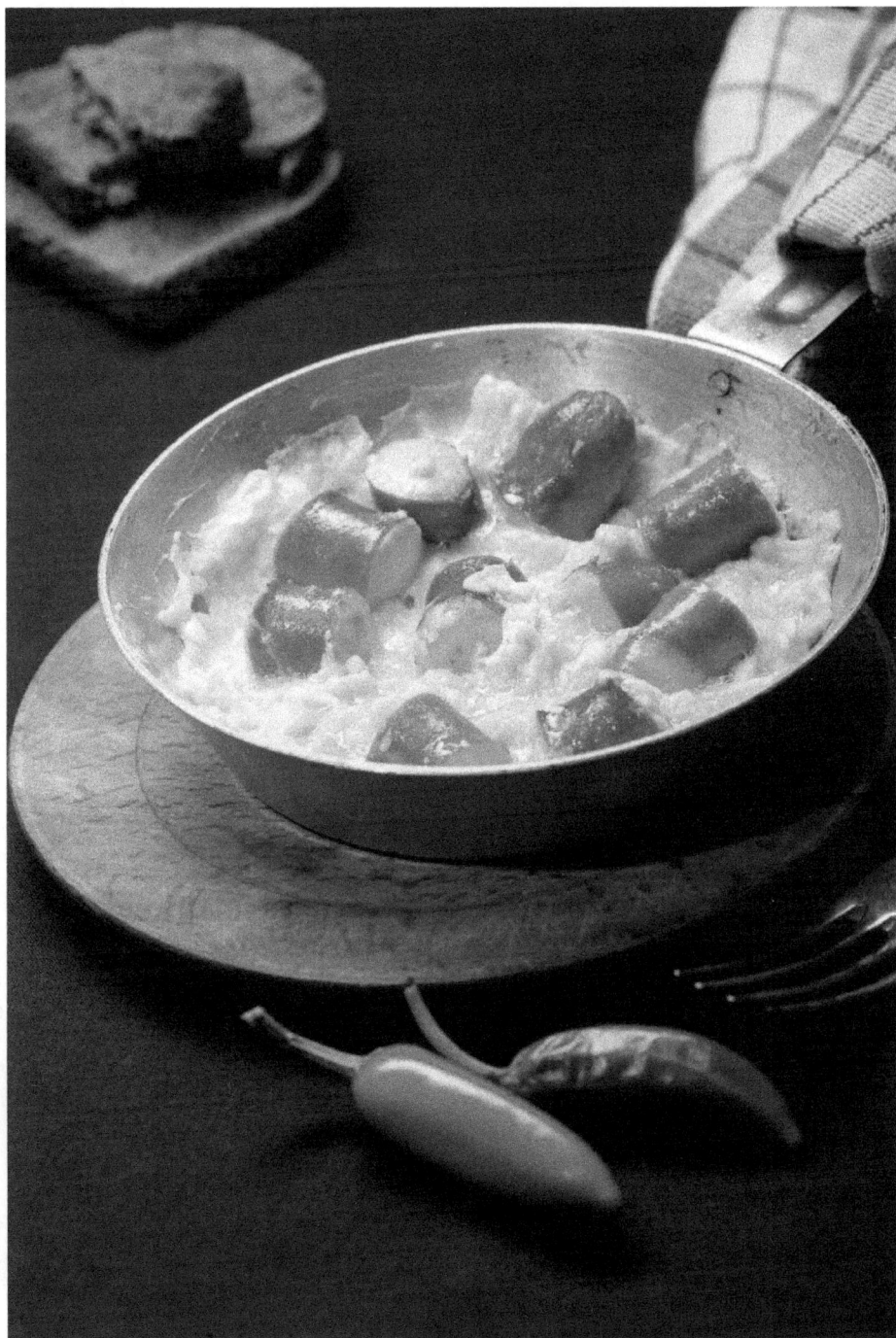

Pear Oatmeal

Servings: 4
Cooking Time: 25 Minutes

Ingredients:
- 1 cup oatmeal
- 1/3 cup milk
- 1 pear, chopped
- 1 teaspoon vanilla extract
- 1 tablespoon Splenda
- 1 teaspoon butter
- ½ teaspoon ground cinnamon
- 1 egg, beaten

Directions:
1. In the big bowl mix up together oatmeal, milk, egg, vanilla extract, Splenda, and ground cinnamon.
2. Melt butter and add it in the oatmeal mixture.
3. Then add chopped pear and stir it well.
4. Transfer the oatmeal mixture in the casserole mold and flatten gently. Cover it with the foil and secure edges.
5. Bake the oatmeal for 25 minutes at 350F.

Nutrition Info:Per Serving:calories 151, fat 3.9, fiber 3.3, carbs 23.6, protein 4.9

Mediterranean Frittata

Servings: 6
Cooking Time: 15 Minutes

Ingredients:

- 9 large eggs, lightly beaten
- 8 kalamata olives, pitted, chopped
- 1/4 cup olive oil
- 1/3 cup parmesan cheese, freshly grated
- 1/3 cup fresh basil, thinly sliced
- 1/2 teaspoon salt
- 1/2 teaspoon pepper
- 1/2 cup onion, chopped
- 1 sweet red pepper, diced
- 1 medium zucchini, cut to 1/2-inch cubes
- 1 package (4 ounce) feta cheese, crumbled

Directions:
1. In a 10-inch oven-proof skillet, heat the olive oil until hot. Add the olives, zucchini, red pepper, and the onions, constantly stirring, until the vegetables are tender.
2. Ina bowl, mix the eggs, feta cheese, basil, salt, and pepper; pour in the skillet with vegetables. Adjust heat to medium-low, cover, and cook for about 10-12 minutes, or until the egg mixture is almost set.
3. Remove from the heat and sprinkle with the parmesan cheese. Transfer to the broiler.

4. With oven door partially open, broil 5 1/2 from the source of heat for about 2-3 minutes or until the top is golden. Cut into wedges.

Nutrition Info:Per Serving:288.5 Cal, 22.8 g total fat (7.8 g sat. fat), 301 mg chol., 656 mg sodium, 5.6 g carb.,1.2 g fiber,3.3g sugar, 15.2 g protein.

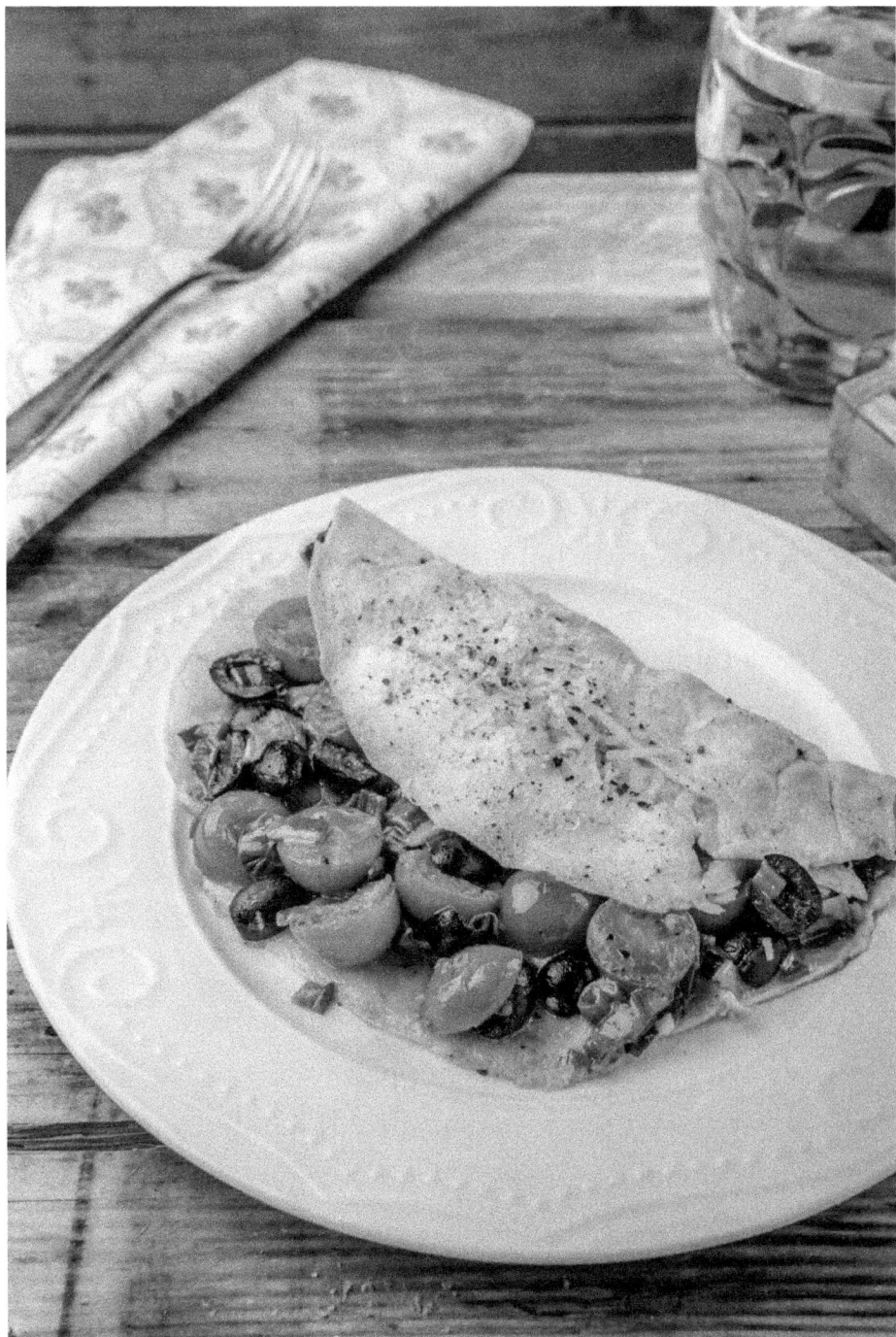

Mediterranean Egg Casserole

Servings: 8

Cooking Time: 50 Minutes

Ingredients:

- 1 1/2 cups (6 ounces) feta cheese, crumbled
- 1 jar (6 ounces) marinated artichoke hearts, drained well, coarsely chopped
- 10 eggs
- 2 cups milk, low-fat
- 2 cups fresh baby spinach, packed, coarsely chopped
- 6 cups whole-wheat baguette, cut into 1-inch cubes
- 1 tablespoon garlic (about 4 cloves), finely chopped
- 1 tablespoon olive oil, extra-virgin
- 1/2 cup red bell pepper, chopped
- 1/2 cup Parmesan cheese, shredded
- 1/2 teaspoon pepper
- 1/2 teaspoon red pepper flakes
- 1/2 teaspoon salt
- 1/3 cup kalamata olives, pitted, halved
- 1/4 cup red onion, chopped
- 1/4 cup tomatoes (sun-dried) in oil, drained, chopped

Directions:

1. Preheat oven to 350F.

2. Grease a 9x13-inch baking dish with olive oil cooking spray.

3. In an 8-inch non-stick pan over medium heat, heat the olive oil. Add the onions, garlic, and bell pepper; cook for about 3 minutes, frequently stirring, until slightly softened. Add the spinach; cook for about 1 minute or until starting to wilt.

4. Layer half of the baguette cubes in the prepared baking dish, then 1 cup of the eta, 1/4 cup Parmesan, the bell pepper mix, artichokes, the olives, and the tomatoes. Top with the remaining baguette cubes and then with the remaining 1/2 cup of feta.

5. In a large mixing bowl, whisk the eggs and the low-fat milk together. Beat in the pepper, salt and the pepper. Pour the mix over the bread layer in the baking dish, slightly pressing down. Sprinkle with the remaining 1/4 cup Parmesan.

6. Bake for about 40-45 minutes, or until the center is set and the top is golden brown. Before serving, let stand for 15 minutes.

Nutrition Info:Per Serving:360 Cal, 21 g total fat (9 g sat. fat), 270 mg chol., 880 mg sodium, 24 g carb.,3 g fiber,7 g sugar, 20 g protein.

Milk Scones

Servings: 4
Cooking Time: 10 Minutes

Ingredients:
- ½ cup wheat flour, whole grain
- 1 teaspoon baking powder
- 1 tablespoon butter, melted
- 1 teaspoon vanilla extract
- 1 egg, beaten
- ¾ teaspoon salt
- 3 tablespoons milk
- 1 teaspoon vanilla sugar

Directions:
1. In the mixing bowl combine together wheat flour, baking powder, butter, vanilla extract, and egg. Add salt and knead the soft and non-sticky dough. Add more flour if needed.
2. Then make the log from the dough and cut it into the triangles.
3. Line the tray with baking paper.
4. Arrange the dough triangles on the baking paper and transfer in the preheat to the 360F oven.
5. Cook the scones for 10 minutes or until they are light brown.

6. After this, chill the scones and brush with milk and sprinkle with vanilla sugar.

Nutrition Info:Per Serving:calories 112, fat 4.4, fiber 0.5, carbs 14.3, protein 3.4

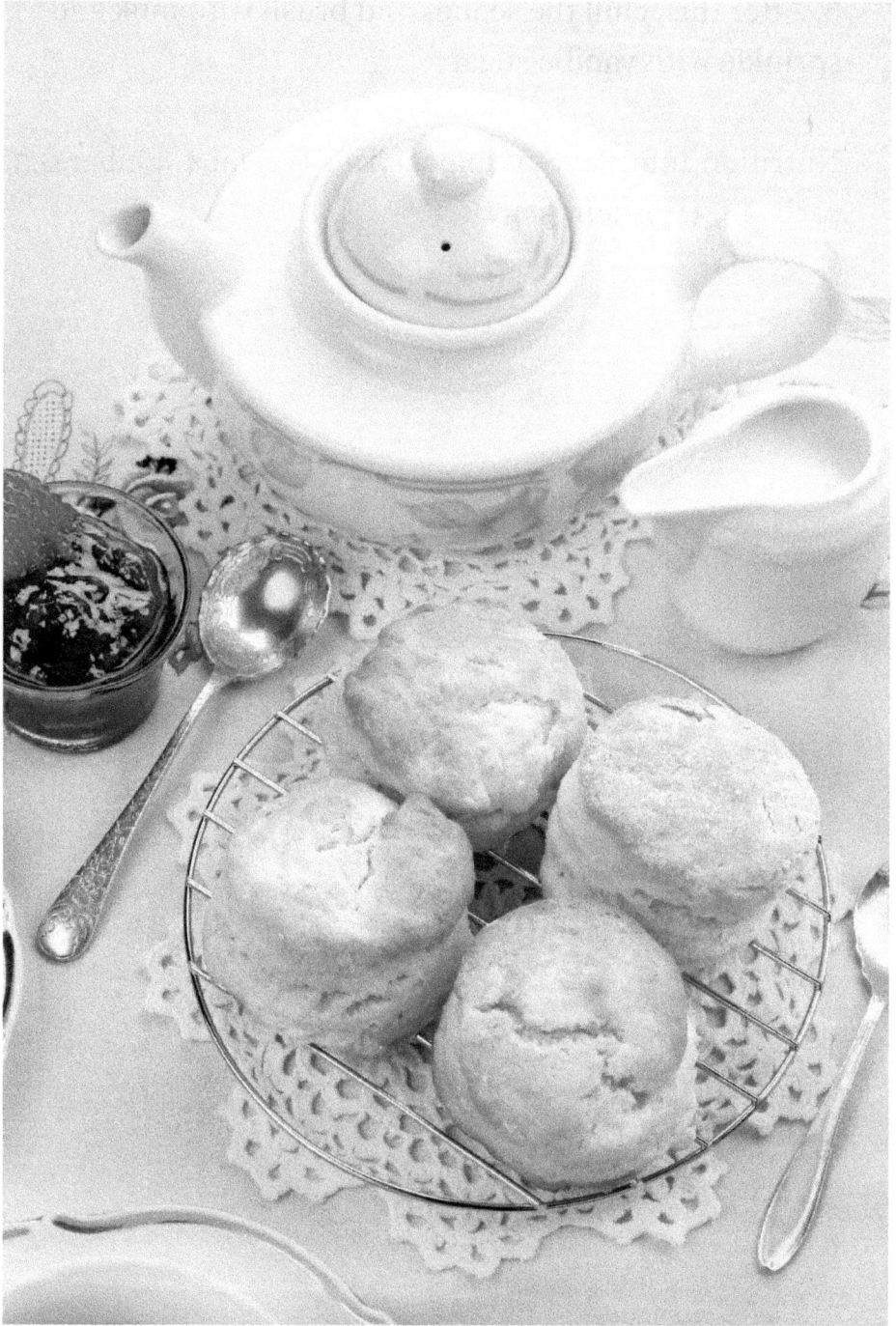

Herbed Eggs And Mushroom Mix

Servings: 4

Cooking Time: 20 Minutes

Ingredients:

- 1 red onion, chopped
- 1 bell pepper, chopped
- 1 tablespoon tomato paste
- 1/3 cup water
- ½ teaspoon of sea salt
- 1 tablespoon butter
- 1 cup cremini mushrooms, chopped
- 1 tablespoon fresh parsley
- 1 tablespoon fresh dill
- 1 teaspoon dried thyme
- ½ teaspoon dried oregano
- ½ teaspoon paprika
- ½ teaspoon chili flakes
- ½ teaspoon garlic powder
- 4 eggs

Directions:

1. Toss butter in the pan and melt it.
2. Then add chopped mushrooms and bell pepper.
3. Roast the vegetables for 5 minutes over the medium heat.
4. After this, add red onion and stir well.

5. Sprinkle the ingredients with garlic powder, chili flakes, dried oregano, and dried thyme. Mix up well

6. After this, add tomato paste and water.

7. Mix up the mixture until it is homogenous.

8. Then add fresh parsley and dill.

9. Cook the mixture for 5 minutes over the medium-high heat with the closed lid.

10. After this, stir the mixture with the help of the spatula well.

11. Crack the eggs over the mixture and close the lid.

12. Cook shakshuka for 10 minutes over the low heat.

Nutrition Info:Per Serving:calories 123, fat 7.5, fiber 1.7, carbs 7.8, protein 7.1 25. Leeks And

Eggs Muffins

Servings: 2

Cooking Time: 20 Minutes

Ingredients:

- 3 eggs, whisked
- ¼ cup baby spinach
- 2 tablespoons leeks, chopped
- 4 tablespoons parmesan, grated
- 2 tablespoons almond milk
- Cooking spray
- 1 small red bell pepper, chopped
- Salt and black pepper to the taste
- 1 tomato, cubed
- 2 tablespoons cheddar cheese, grated

Directions:

1. In a bowl, combine the eggs with the milk, salt, pepper and the rest of the ingredients except the cooking spray and whisk well.

2. Grease a muffin tin with the cooking spray and divide the eggs mixture in each muffin mould.

3. Bake at 380 degrees F for 20 minutes and serve them for breakfast.

Nutrition Info: calories 308, fat 19.4, fiber 1.7, carbs 8.7, protein 24.4

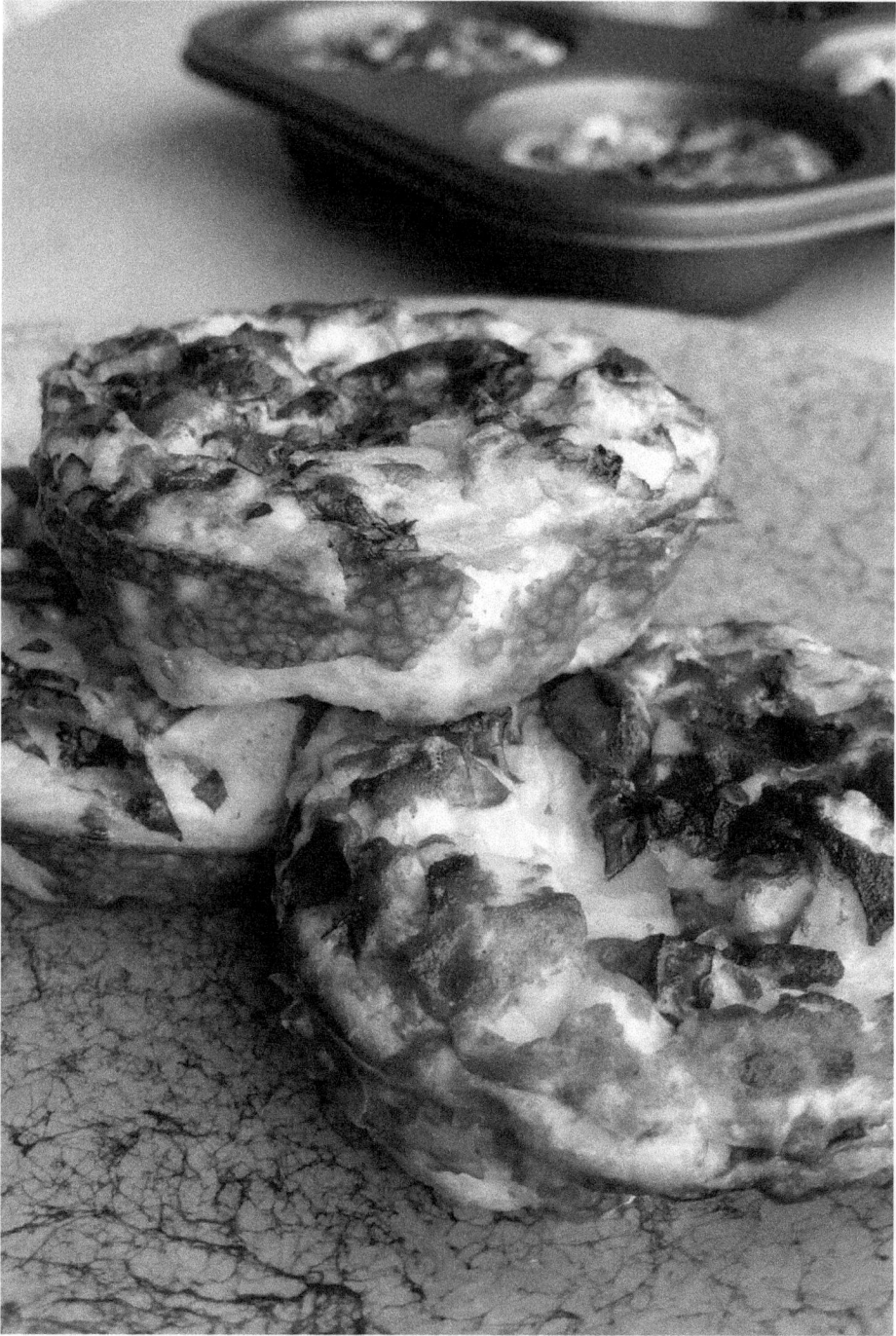

Mango And Spinach Bowls

Servings: 4
Cooking Time: 0 Minutes

Ingredients:
- 1 cup baby arugula
- 1 cup baby spinach, chopped
- 1 mango, peeled and cubed
- 1 cup strawberries, halved
- 1 tablespoon hemp seeds
- 1 cucumber, sliced
- 1 tablespoon lime juice
- 1 tablespoon tahini paste
- 1 tablespoon water

Directions:
1. In a salad bowl, mix the arugula with the rest of the ingredients except the tahini and the water and toss.
2. In a small bowl, combine the tahini with the water, whisk well, add to the salad, toss, divide into small bowls and serve for breakfast.

Nutrition Info: calories 211, fat 4.5, fiber 6.5, carbs 10.2, protein 3.5

Veggie Quiche

Servings: 8

Cooking Time: 55 Minutes

Ingredients:

- ½ cup sun-dried tomatoes, chopped
- 1 prepared pie crust
- 2 tablespoons avocado oil
- 1 yellow onion, chopped
- 2 garlic cloves, minced
- 2 cups spinach, chopped
- 1 red bell pepper, chopped
- ¼ cup kalamata olives, pitted and sliced
- 1 teaspoon parsley flakes
- 1 teaspoon oregano, dried
- 1/3 cup feta cheese, crumbled
- 4 eggs, whisked
- 1 and ½ cups almond milk
- 1 cup cheddar cheese, shredded
- Salt and black pepper to the taste

Directions:

1. Heat up a pan with the oil over medium-high heat, add the garlic and onion and sauté for 3 minutes.

2. Add the bell pepper and sauté for 3 minutes more.

3. Add the olives, parsley, spinach, oregano, salt and pepper and cook everything for 5 minutes.

4. Add tomatoes and the cheese, toss and take off the heat.

5. Arrange the pie crust in a pie plate, pour the spinach and tomatoes mix inside and spread.

6. In a bowl, mix the eggs with salt, pepper, the milk and half of the cheese, whisk and pour over the mixture in the pie crust.

7. Sprinkle the remaining cheese on top and bake at 375 degrees F for 40 minutes.

8. Cool the quiche down, slice and serve for breakfast.

Nutrition Info: calories 211, fat 14.4, fiber 1.4, carbs 12.5, protein 8.6

Tuna And Cheese Bake

Servings: 4

Cooking Time: 15 Minutes

Ingredients:

- 10 ounces canned tuna, drained and flaked
- 4 eggs, whisked
- ½ cup feta cheese, shredded
- 1 tablespoon chives, chopped
- 1 tablespoon parsley, chopped
- Salt and black pepper to the taste
- 3 teaspoons olive oil

Directions:

1. Grease a baking dish with the oil, add the tuna and the rest of the ingredients except the cheese, toss and bake at 370 degrees F for 15 minutes.
2. Sprinkle the cheese on top, leave the mix aside for 5 minutes, slice and serve for breakfast.

Nutrition Info: calories 283, fat 14.2, fiber 5.6, carbs 12.1, protein 6.4

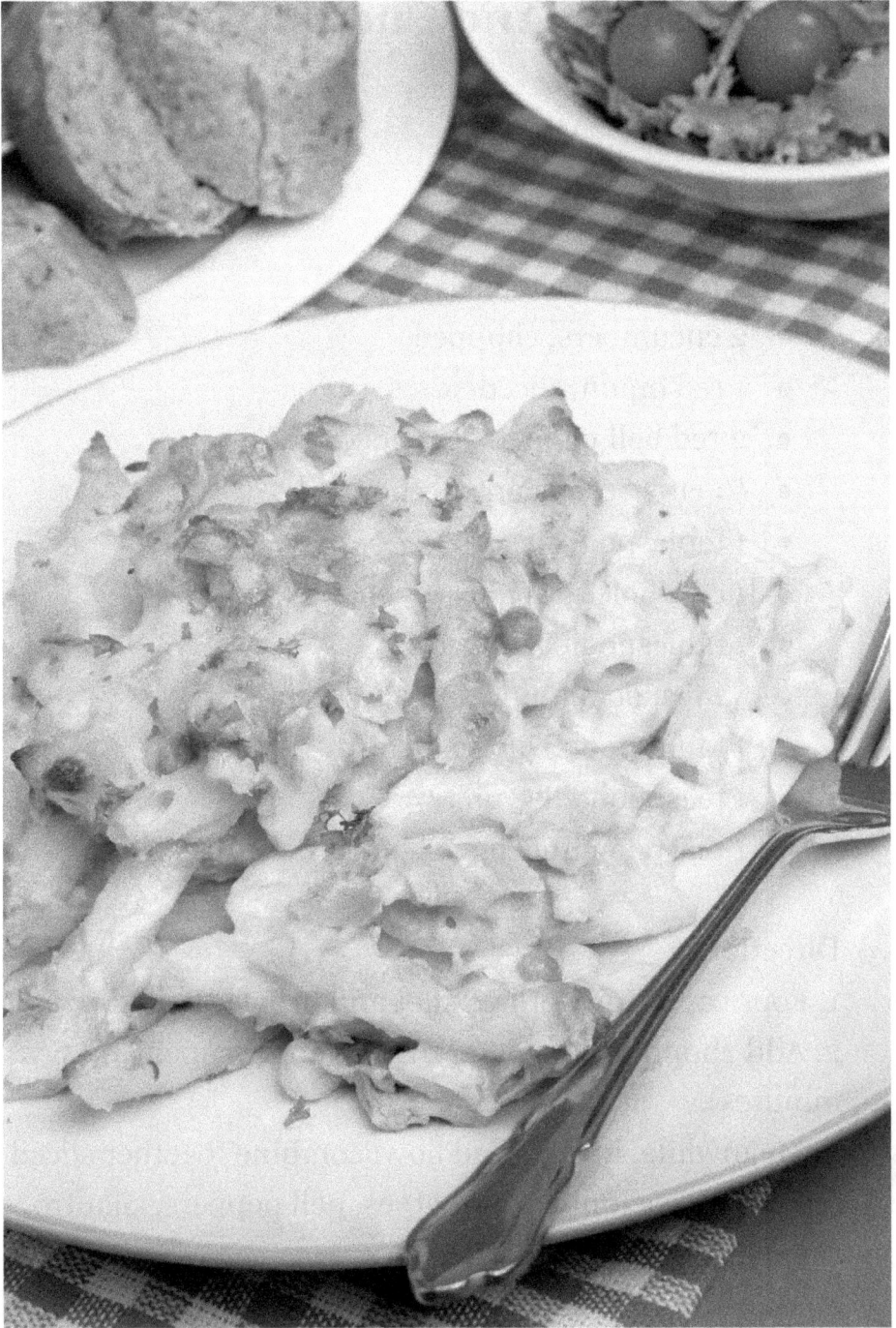

Tomato And Cucumber Salad

Servings: 4
Cooking Time: 5 Minutes

Ingredients:
- 3 tomatoes, chopped
- 2 cucumbers, chopped
- 1 red onion, sliced
- 2 red bell peppers, chopped
- ¼ cup fresh cilantro, chopped
- 1 tablespoon capers
- 1 oz whole-grain bread, chopped
- 1 tablespoon canola oil
- ½ teaspoon minced garlic
- 1 tablespoon Dijon mustard
- 1 teaspoon olive oil
- 1 teaspoon lime juice

Directions:
1. Pour canola oil in the skillet and bring it to boil.
2. Add chopped bread and roast it until crunchy (3-5 minutes).
3. Meanwhile, in the salad bowl combine together sliced red onion, cucumbers, tomatoes, bell peppers, cilantro, capers, and mix up gently.
4. Make the dressing: mix up together lime juice, olive oil, Dijon mustard, and minced garlic.

5. Pour the dressing over the salad and stir it directly before serving.

Nutrition Info:Per Serving:calories 136, fat 5.7, fiber 4.1, carbs 20.2, protein 4.1

Cream Olive Muffins

Servings: 6

Cooking Time: 20 Minutes

Ingredients:

- ½ cup quinoa, cooked
- 2 oz Feta cheese, crumbled
- 2 eggs, beaten
- 3 kalamata olives, chopped
- ¾ cup heavy cream
- 1 tomato, chopped
- 1 teaspoon butter, softened
- 1 tablespoon wheat flour, whole grain
- ½ teaspoon salt

Directions:

1. In the mixing bowl whisk eggs and add Feta cheese.
2. Then add chopped tomato and heavy cream.
3. After this, add wheat flour, salt, and quinoa.
4. Then add kalamata olives and mix up the ingredients with the help of the spoon.
5. Brush the muffin molds with the butter from inside.
6. Transfer quinoa mixture in the muffin molds and flatten it with the help of the spatula or spoon if needed.
7. Cook the muffins in the preheated to 355F oven for 20 minutes.

Nutrition Info:Per Serving:calories 165, fat 10.8, fiber 1.2, carbs 11.5, protein 5.8

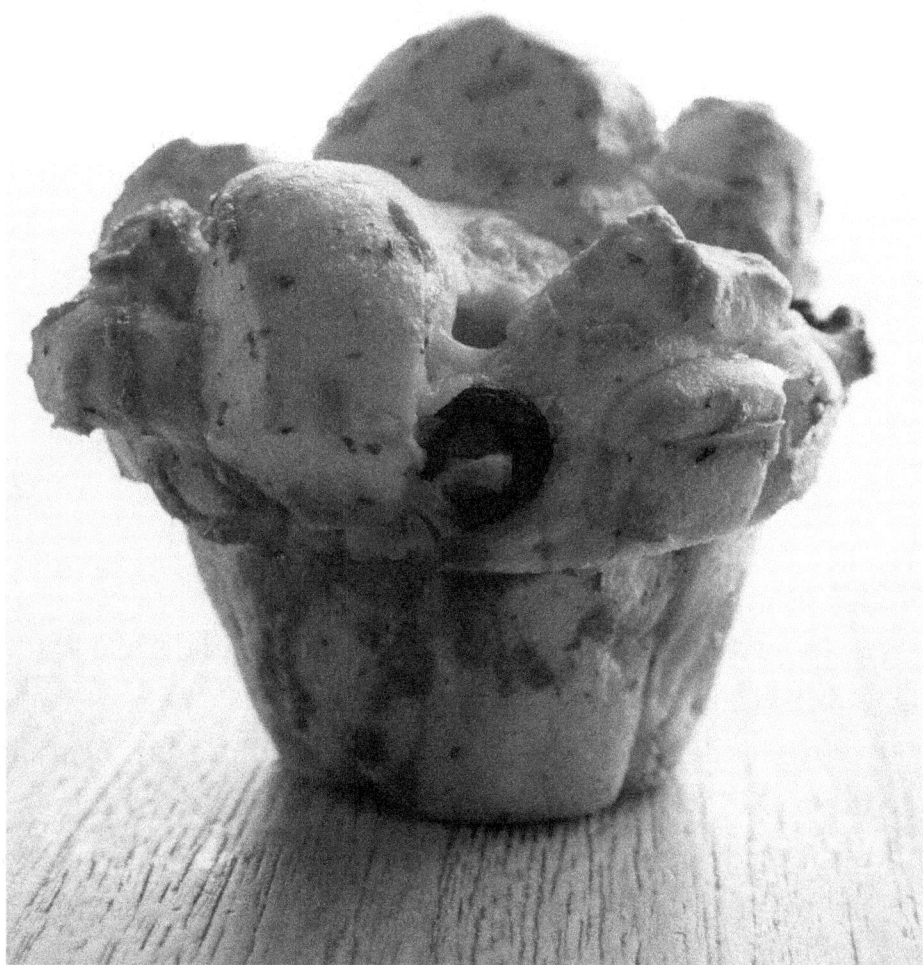

Roasted Asparagus With Prosciutto And Poached Egg

Servings: 4

Cooking Time: 25 Minutes

Ingredients:

- 1 bunch fresh asparagus, trimmed
- 1 tablespoon extra-virgin olive oil
- 4 eggs
- 2 ounces minced prosciutto
- 1/2 lemon, zested and juiced
- 1 tablespoon olive oil
- 1 pinch salt
- 1 pinch ground black pepper
- 1 teaspoon distilled white vinegar
- Ground black pepper

Directions:

1. Preheat oven to 425F or 220C.
2. In a baking dish, place the asparagus and drizzle with the extra-virgin olive oil.
3. In a skillet, heat the olive oil over medium-low heat; add the prosciutto and cook for about 3-4 minutes, stirring, until golden and rendered. Sprinkle over the asparagus in the baking dish and season with black pepper; toss to coat.

4. Roast for 10 minutes, toss, return to the oven, and continue roasting for 5 minutes or until the asparagus are tender yet firm to the bite.

5. Fill a large saucepan with about 2-3 inches of water; bring to a boil over high heat. When boiling, reduce the heat to low; pour in the vinegar and a pinch of salt. Crack an egg into a small bowl, then gently slip the egg into the water. Repeat with the remaining eggs. Poach the eggs for about 4-6 minutes or until the whites are firm and the yolks are thick but not hard. With a slotted spoon, remove the eggs, dab the spoon on a clean kitchen towel to remove excess water from the eggs, and transfer to a warm plate.

6. Drizzle the asparagus with the lemon juice and transfer divide between 2 plates. Top each asparagus bed with the 2 poached eggs, sprinkle with a pinch of lemon zest, and season with black pepper; serve.

Nutrition Info:Per Serving:163 Cal, 12.3 g total fat (2.7 g sat. fat), 171 mg chol., 273 mg sodium, 4.3 g carb., 1.9 g fiber, 10.4 g protein.

Figs Oatmeal

Servings: 5
Cooking Time: 20 Minutes

Ingredients:
- 2 cups oatmeal
- 1 ½ cup milk
- 1 tablespoon butter
- 3 figs, chopped
- 1 tablespoon honey

Directions:
1. Pour milk in the saucepan.
2. Add oatmeal and close the lid.
3. Cook the oatmeal for 15 minutes over the medium-low heat.
4. Then add chopped figs and honey.
5. Add butter and mix up the oatmeal well.
6. Cook it for 5 minutes more.
7. Close the lid and let the cooked breakfast rest for 10 minutes before serving.

Nutrition Info:Per Serving:calories 222, fat 6, fiber 4.4, carbs 36.5, protein 7.1 33.

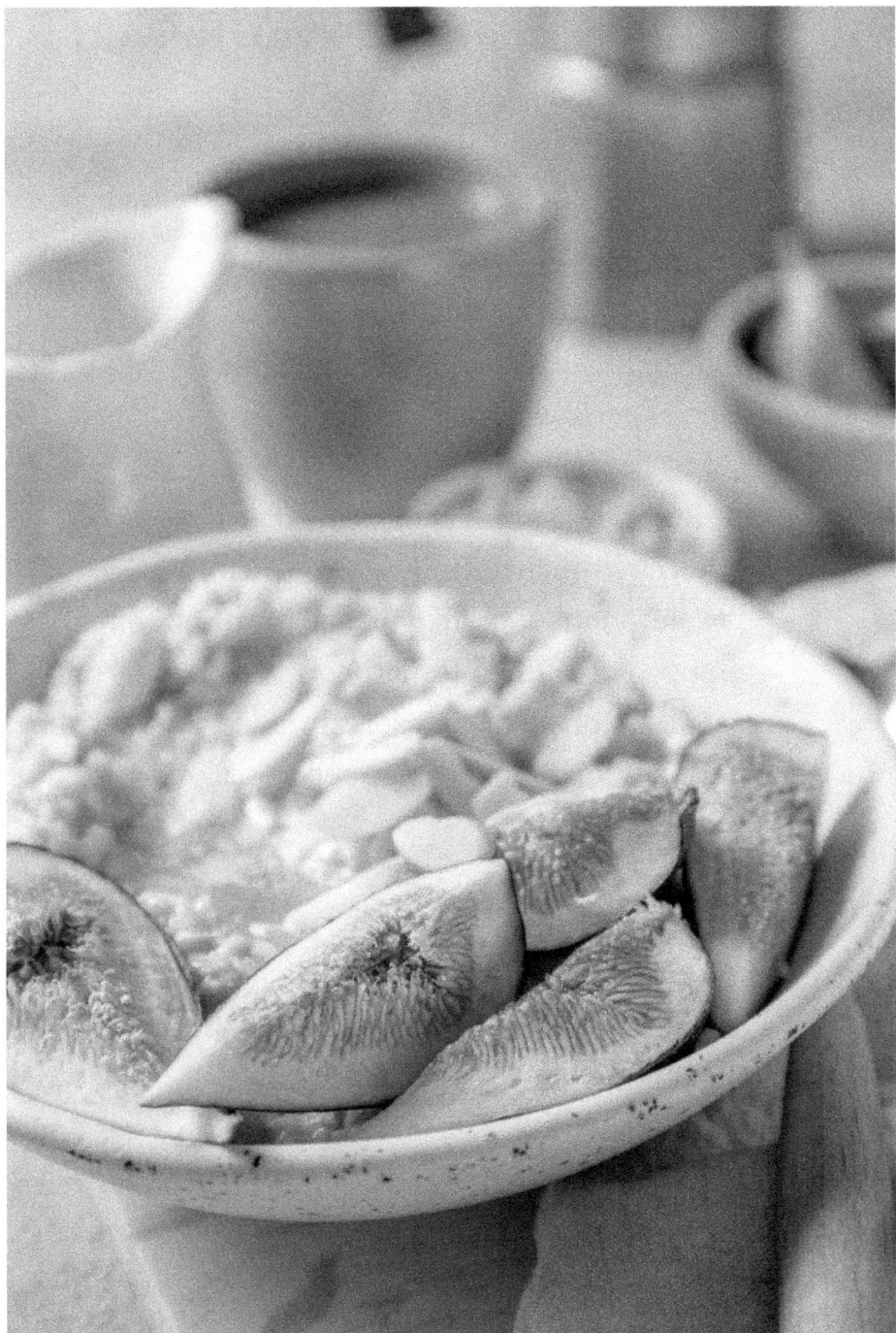

Mediterranean Freezer Breakfast Wraps

Servings: 4

Cooking Time: 3 Minutes

Ingredients:

- 1 cup spinach leaves, fresh, chopped
- 1 tablespoon water or low-fat milk
- 1/2 teaspoon garlic-chipotle seasoning or your preferred seasoning 4 eggs, beaten
- 4 pieces (8-inch) whole-wheat tortillas
- 4 tablespoons tomato chutney (or dried tomatoes, chopped or canned tomatoes)
- 4 tablespoons feta cheese, crumbled (or goat cheese)
- Optional: prosciutto, chopped or bacon, cooked, crumbled
- Salt and pepper, to taste

Directions:

1. In a mixing bowl, whisk the eggs, water or milk, and seasoning together.
2. Heat a skillet with a little olive oil; pour the eggs and scramble for about 3-4 minutes, or until just cooked.
3. Lay the tortillas in a clean surface; divide the eggs between them, arranging the scrambled eggs in a line and leaving the tortilla edges free to fold later.

4. Top the egg layer with about 1 tablespoon of cheese, 1 tablespoon tomatoes, and 1/4 cup spinach. If using, layer with prosciutto or bacon.

5. In a burrito-style, roll up the tortillas, folding both of the ends in the

process.

6. In a panini maker or a clean skillet, cook for about 1 minute, turning once, until the tortilla wraps are crisp and brown; serve.

Nutrition Info:Per Serving:450 Cal, 15 g total fat (5 g sat. fat), 220 mg chol., 1, 280 mg sodium, 960 mg pot., 64 g carb.,6 g fiber,20 g sugar, 17 g protein.

Cheesy Olives Bread

Servings: 10

Cooking Time: 30 Minutes

Ingredients:

- 4 cups whole-wheat flour
- 3 tablespoons oregano, chopped
- 2 teaspoons dry yeast
- ¼ cup olive oil
- 1 and ½ cups black olives, pitted and sliced
- 1 cup water
- ½ cup feta cheese, crumbled

Directions:

1. In a bowl, mix the flour with the water, the yeast and the oil, stir and knead your dough very well.

2. Put the dough in a bowl, cover with plastic wrap and keep in a warm place for 1 hour.

3. Divide the dough into 2 bowls and stretch each ball really well.

4. Add the rest of the ingredients on each ball and tuck them inside well kneading the dough again.

5. Flatten the balls a bit and leave them aside for 40 minutes more.

6. Transfer the balls to a baking sheet lined with parchment paper, make a small slit in each and bake at 425 degrees F for 30 minutes.

7. Serve the bread as a Mediterranean breakfast.

Nutrition Info: calories 251, fat 7.3, fiber 2.1, carbs 39.7, protein 6.7

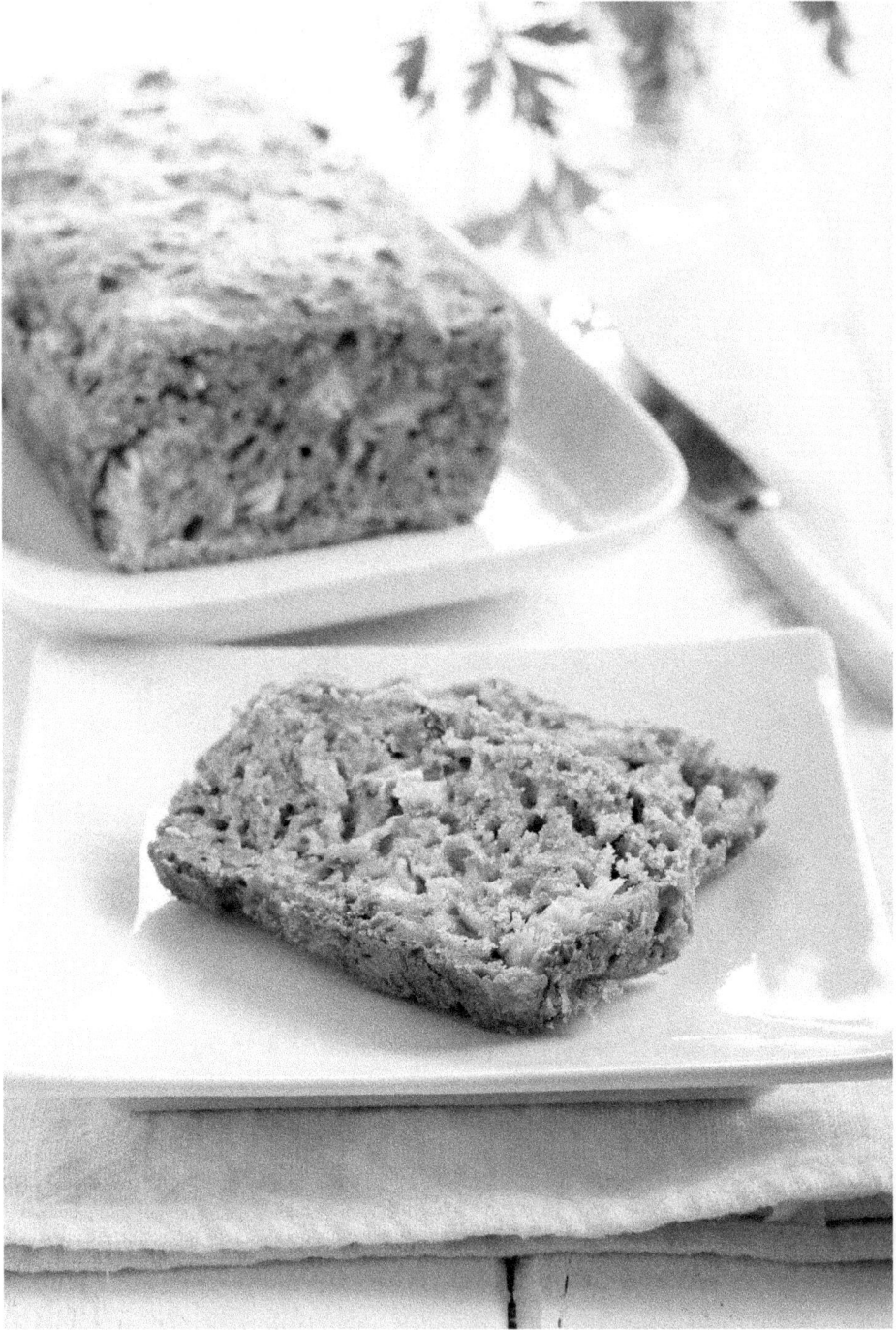

Scrambled Eggs

Servings: 2

Cooking Time: 10 Minutes

Ingredients:

- 1 yellow bell pepper, chopped
- 8 cherry tomatoes, cubed
- 2 spring onions, chopped
- 1 tablespoon olive oil
- 1 tablespoon capers, drained
- 2 tablespoons black olives, pitted and sliced
- 4 eggs
- A pinch of salt and black pepper
- ¼ teaspoon oregano, dried
- 1 tablespoon parsley, chopped

Directions:

1. Heat up a pan with the oil over medium-high heat, add the bell pepper and spring onions and sauté for 3 minutes.
2. Add the tomatoes, capers and the olives and sauté for 2 minutes more.
3. Crack the eggs into the pan, add salt, pepper and the oregano and scramble for 5 minutes more.
4. Divide the scramble between plates, sprinkle the parsley on top and serve.

Nutrition Info: calories 249, fat 17, fiber 3.2, carbs 13.3, protein 13.5

Paprika Salmon Toast

Servings: 2

Cooking Time: 3 Minutes

Ingredients:
- 4 whole grain bread slices
- 2 oz smoked salmon, sliced
- 2 teaspoons cream cheese
- 1 teaspoon fresh dill, chopped
- ½ teaspoon lemon juice
- ½ teaspoon paprika
- 4 lettuce leaves
- 1 cucumber, sliced

Directions:

1. Toast the bread in the toaster (1-2 minutes totally).

2. In the bowl, mix up together fresh dill, cream cheese, lemon juice, and paprika.

3. Then spread the toasts with the cream cheese mixture.

4. Slice the smoked salmon and place it on 2 bread slices.

5. Add sliced cucumber and lettuce leaves.

6. Top the lettuce with remaining bread toasts and pin with the toothpick.

Nutrition Info:Per Serving:calories 202, fat 4.7, fiber 5.1, carbs 31.5, protein 12.7

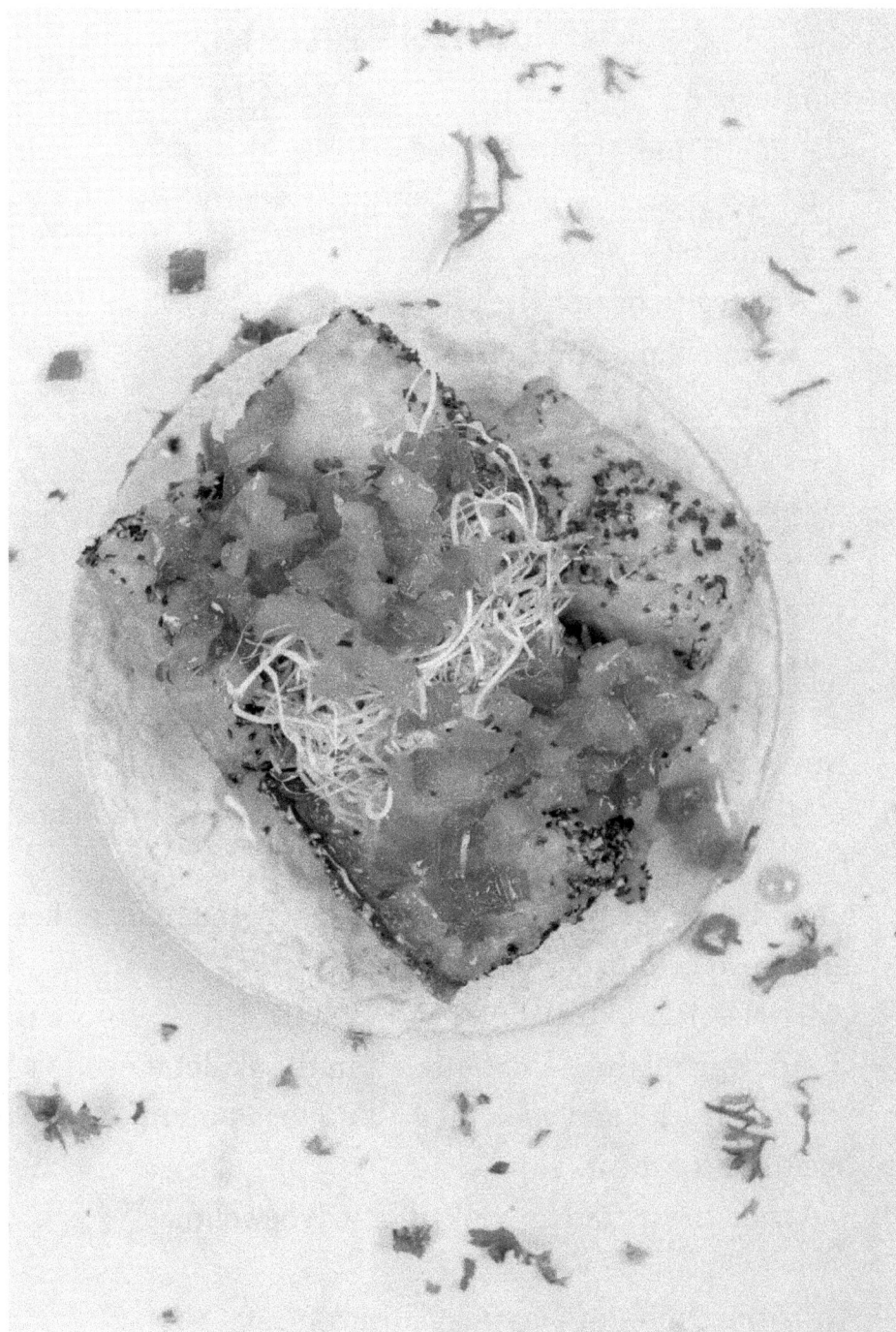

Creamy Frittata

Servings: 4
Cooking Time: 15 Minutes

Ingredients:

- 5 eggs, beaten
- 1 poblano chile, chopped, raw
- 1 oz scallions, chopped
- 1/3 cup heavy cream
- ½ teaspoon butter
- ½ teaspoon salt
- ½ teaspoon chili flakes
- 1 tablespoon fresh cilantro, chopped

Directions:

1. Mix up together eggs with heavy cream and whisk until homogenous.
2. Add chopped poblano chile, scallions, salt, chili flakes, and fresh cilantro.
3. Toss butter in the skillet and melt it.
4. Add egg mixture and flatten it in the skillet if needed.
5. Close the lid and cook the frittata for 15 minutes over the medium-low heat.
6. When the frittata is cooked, it will be solid.

Nutrition Info:Per Serving:calories 131, fat 10.4, fiber 0.2, carbs 1.3, protein 8.2

Egg And Pepper Bake

Servings: 4

Cooking Time: 28 Minutes

Ingredients:

- 2 eggs, beaten
- 1 red bell pepper, chopped
- 1 chili pepper, chopped
- ½ red onion, diced
- 1 teaspoon canola oil
- ½ teaspoon salt
- 1 teaspoon paprika
- 1 tablespoon fresh cilantro, chopped
- 1 garlic clove, diced
- 1 teaspoon butter, softened
- ¼ teaspoon chili flakes

Directions:

1. Brush the casserole mold with canola oil and pour beaten eggs inside.
2. After this, toss the butter in the skillet and melt it over the medium heat.
3. Add chili pepper and red bell pepper.
4. After this, add red onion and cook the vegetables for 7-8 minutes over the medium heat. Stir them from time to time.
5. Transfer the vegetables in the casserole mold.

6. Add salt, paprika, cilantro, diced garlic, and chili flakes. Stir gently with the help of a spatula to get a homogenous mixture.

7. Bake the casserole for 20 minutes at 355F in the oven.

8. Then chill the meal well and cut into servings. Transfer the casserole in the serving plates with the help of the spatula.

Nutrition Info:Per Serving:calories 68, fat 4.5, fiber 1, carbs 4.4, protein 3.4 39. Mediterranean

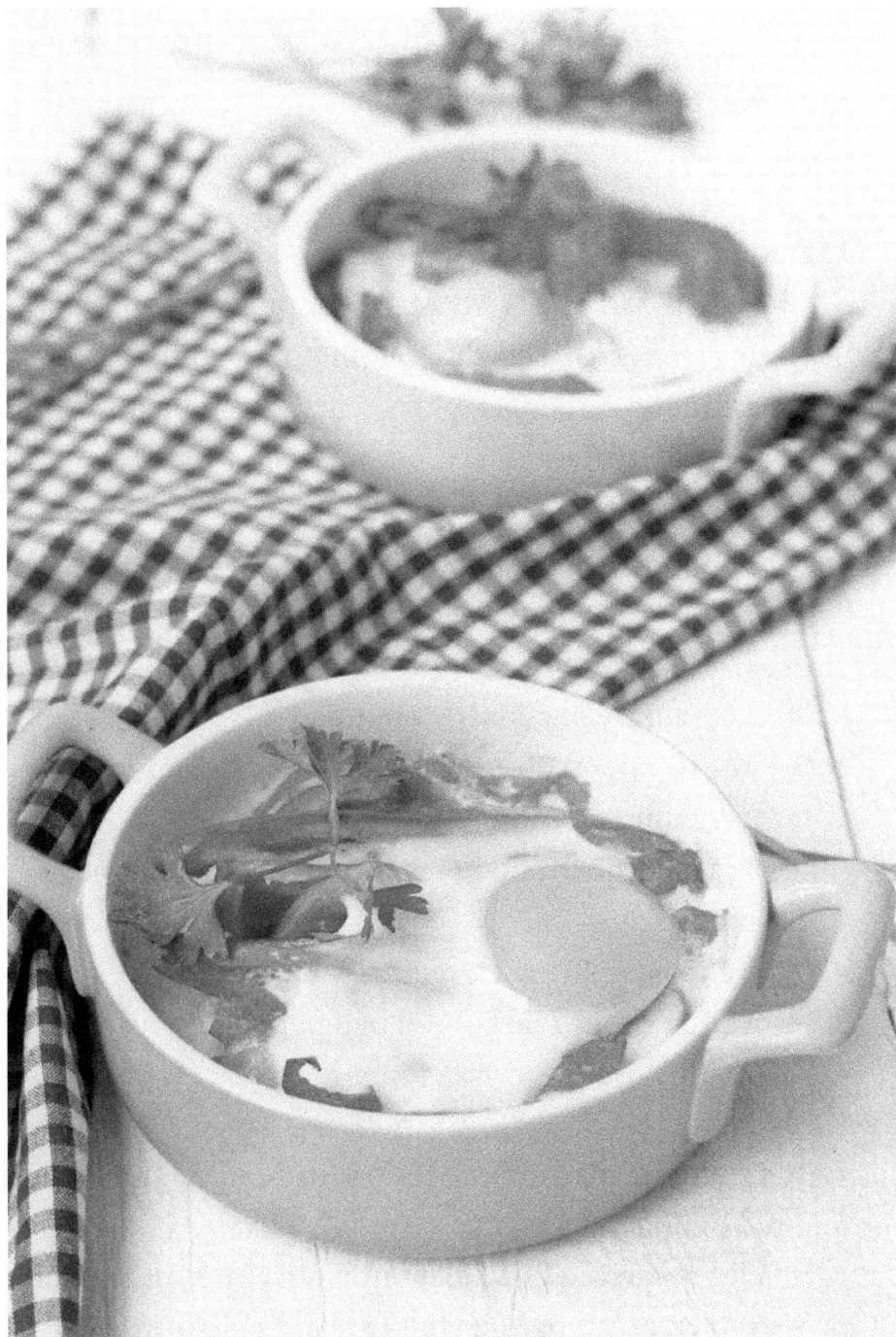

Chicken Salad Pitas

Servings: 6

Cooking Time: 15 Minutes

Ingredients:

- 6 pieces (6-inch) whole-wheat pitas, cut into halves
- 6 slices (1/8-inch-thick) tomato, cut into halves
- 1 can (15-ounce) chickpeas (garbanzo beans), no-salt-added, rinsed, drained
- 3 cups chicken, cooked, chopped
- 2 tablespoons lemon juice
- 12 Bibb lettuce leaves
- 1/4 teaspoon red pepper, crushed
- 1/4 cup fresh cilantro, chopped
- 1/2 teaspoon ground cumin
- 1/2 cup red onion, diced
- 1/2 cup (about 20 small) green olives, chopped, pitted
- 1 cup Greek yogurt, plain, whole-milk
- 1 cup (about 1 large) red bell pepper, chopped

Directions:

1. In a small bowl, combine the yogurt, lemon juice, cumin, and red pepper; set aside.

2. In a large mixing bowl, combine the chicken, red bell pepper, olives, red onion, cilantro, and chickpeas. Add the

yogurt mixture into the chicken mixture; gently toss to coat.

3. Line each pita half with 1 lettuce leaf and then with 1 tomato slice. Fill each pita half with 1/2 cup of the chicken mixture.

Nutrition Info:Per Serving:404 Cal, 10.2 g total fat (3.8 g sat. fat, 1.5 g poly. Fat, 4 g mono), 66 mg chol., 575 mg sodium, 46.4 g carb.,6 g fiber,33.6 g protein.

Raspberries And Yogurt Smoothie

Servings: 2

Cooking Time: 0 Minutes

Ingredients:

- 2 cups raspberries
- ½ cup Greek yogurt
- ½ cup almond milk
- ½ teaspoon vanilla extract

Directions:

1. In your blender, combine the raspberries with the milk, vanilla and the yogurt, pulse well, divide into 2 glasses and serve for breakfast.

Nutrition Info: calories 245, fat 9.5, fiber 2.3, carbs 5.6, protein 1.6

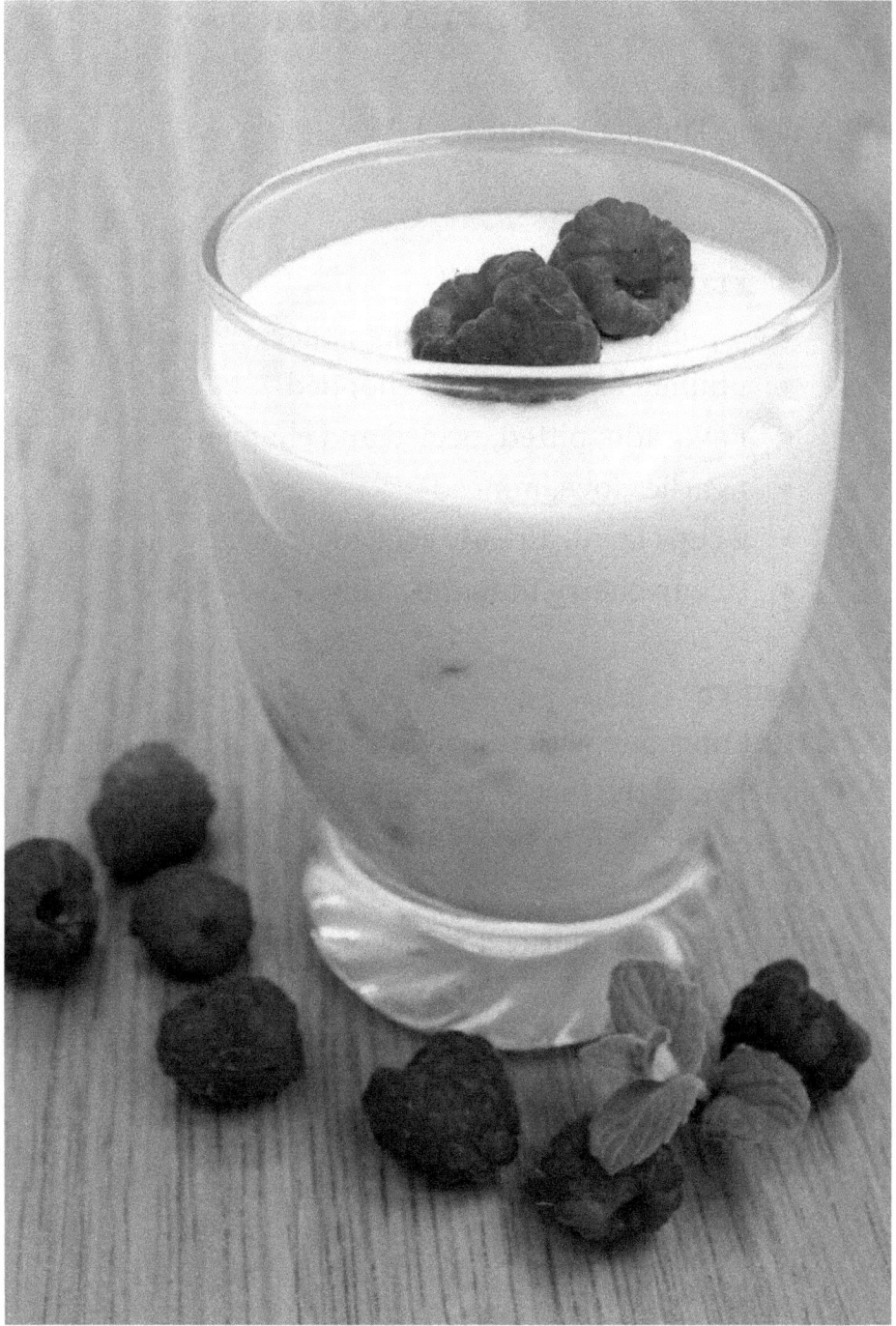

Farro Salad

Servings: 2
Cooking Time: 4 Minutes

Ingredients:
- 1 tablespoon olive oil
- A pinch of salt and black pepper
- 1 bunch baby spinach, chopped
- 1 avocado, pitted, peeled and chopped
- 1 garlic clove, minced
- 2 cups farro, already cooked
- ½ cup cherry tomatoes, cubed

Directions:
1. Heat up a pan with the oil over medium heat, add the spinach, and the rest of the ingredients, toss, cook for 4 minutes, divide into bowls and serve.

Nutrition Info: calories 157, fat 13.7, fiber 5.5, carbs 8.6, protein 3.6

Chili Avocado Scramble

Servings: 4

Cooking Time: 15 Minutes

Ingredients:

- 4 eggs, beaten
- 1 white onion, diced
- 1 tablespoon avocado oil
- 1 avocado, finely chopped
- ½ teaspoon chili flakes
- 1 oz Cheddar cheese, shredded
- ½ teaspoon salt
- 1 tablespoon fresh parsley

Directions:

1. Pour avocado oil in the skillet and bring it to boil.
2. Then add diced onion and roast it until it is light brown.
3. Meanwhile, mix up together chili flakes, beaten eggs, and salt.
4. Pour the egg mixture over the cooked onion and cook the mixture for 1 minute over the medium heat.
5. After this, scramble the eggs well with the help of the fork or spatula. Cook the eggs until they are solid but soft.
6. After this, add chopped avocado and shredded cheese.
7. Stir the scramble well and transfer in the serving plates.
8. Sprinkle the meal with fresh parsley.

Nutrition Info:Per Serving:calories 236, fat 20.1, fiber 4, carbs 7.4, protein 8.6

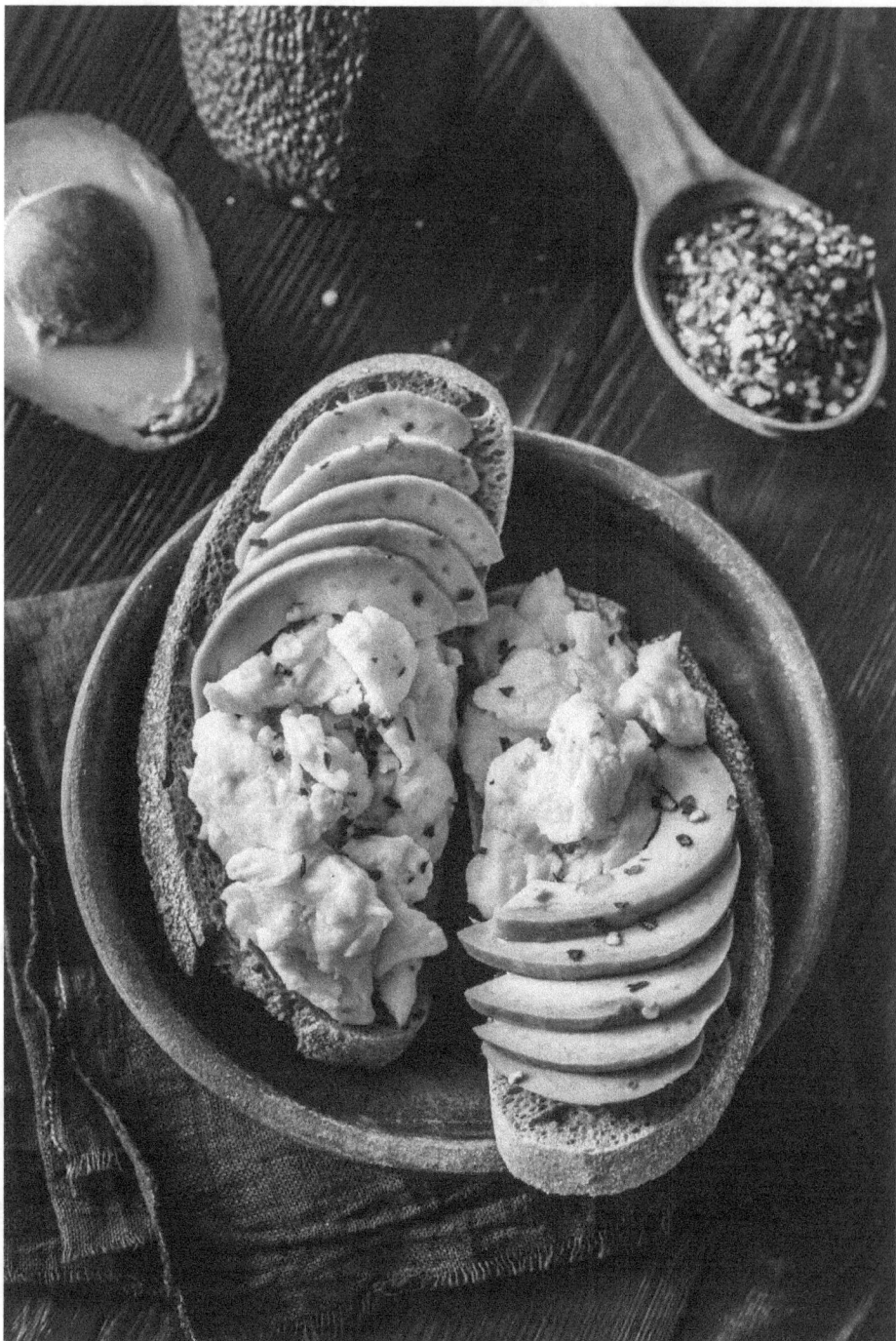

Tapioca Pudding

Servings: 3

Cooking Time: 15 Minutes

Ingredients:

- ¼ cup pearl tapioca
- ¼ cup maple syrup
- 2 cups almond milk
- ½ cup coconut flesh, shredded
- 1 and ½ teaspoon lemon juice

Directions:

1. In a pan, combine the milk with the tapioca and the rest of the ingredients, bring to a simmer over medium heat, and cook for 15 minutes.
2. Divide the mix into bowls, cool it down and serve for breakfast.

Nutrition Info: calories 361, fat 28.5, fiber 2.7, carbs 28.3, protein 2.8

Feta And Eggs Mix

Servings: 4

Cooking Time: 5 Minutes

Ingredients:

- 4 eggs, beaten
- ½ teaspoon ground black pepper
- 2 oz Feta, scrambled
- ½ teaspoon salt
- 1 teaspoon butter
- 1 teaspoon fresh parsley, chopped

Directions:

1. Melt butter in the skillet and add beaten eggs.
2. Then add parsley, salt, and scrambled eggs. Cook the eggs for 1 minute over the high heat.
3. Add ground black pepper and scramble eggs with the help of the fork.
4. Cook the eggs for 3 minutes over the medium-high heat.

Nutrition Info:Per Serving:calories 110, fat 8.4, fiber 0.1, carbs 1.1, protein 7.6

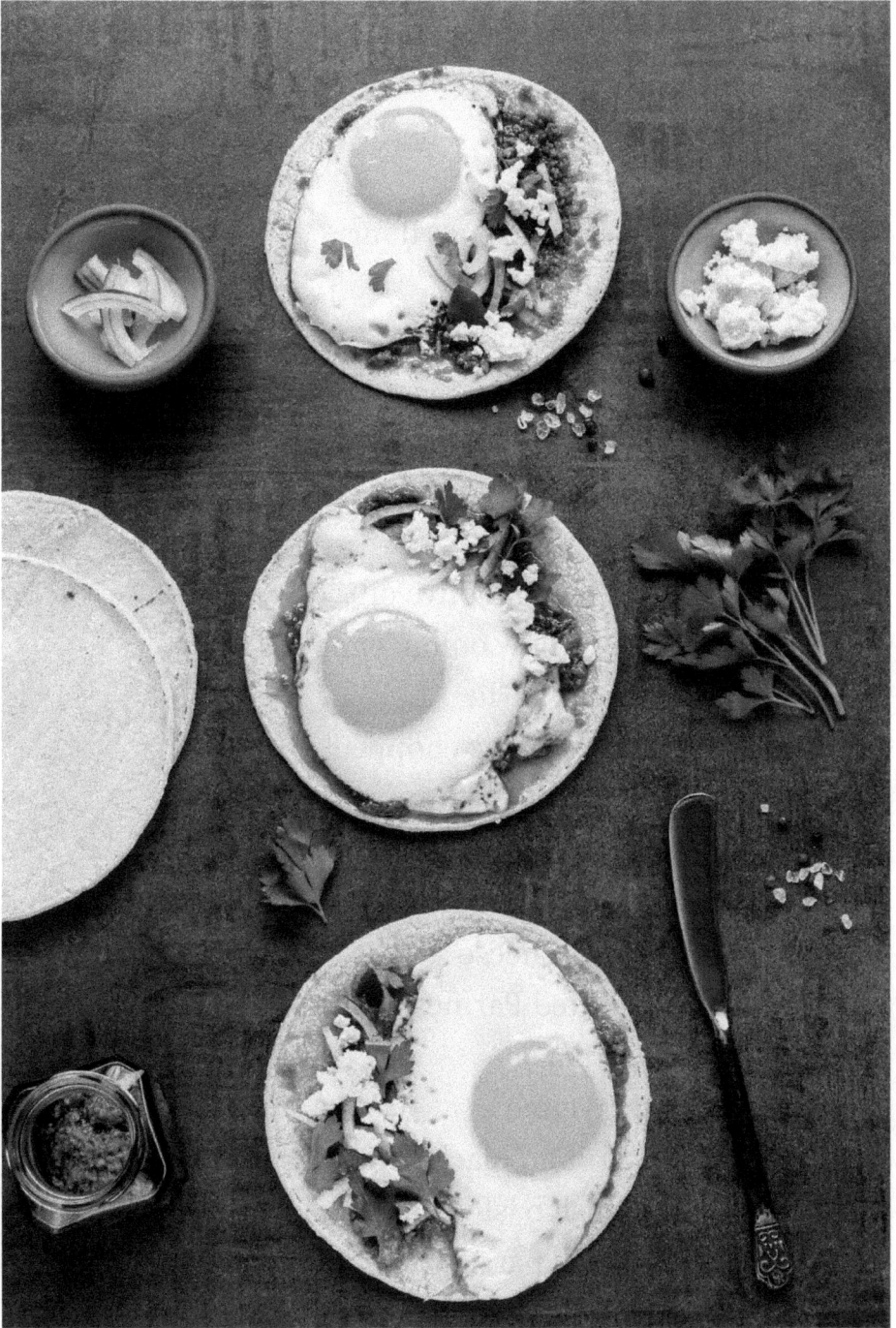

Mediterranean Breakfast Quiche

Servings: ⅛ Quiche

Cooking Time: 1 Hour

Ingredients:

- 11/2 cups all-purpose flour
- 1 tsp. dried oregano
- 1/2 tsp. garlic powder
- 2 tsp. salt
- 5 TB. cold butter
- 3 TB. vegetable shortening
- 1/4 cup ice water
- 3 TB. extra-virgin olive oil
- 1 medium yellow onion, chopped
- 1 TB. minced garlic
- 4 stalks asparagus, chopped
- 2 cups spinach, chopped
- 4 large eggs
- 1/2 cup heavy cream
- 1 cup ricotta cheese
- 1/3 cup grated Parmesan cheese
- 1 tsp. paprika
- 1/2 tsp. cayenne
- 1/2 tsp. ground black pepper
- 1/4 cup fresh basil, chopped
- 1/4 cup fresh parsley, chopped
- 1/3 cup sun-dried tomatoes, chopped

Directions:

1. In a food processor fitted with a chopping blade, pulse together 11/2 cups all-purpose flour, oregano, garlic powder, and 1/2 teaspoon salt five times.

2. Add cold butter and vegetable shortening, and pulse for 1 minute or until mixture resembles coarse meal.

3. Continue to pulse while adding ice water, about 1 minute. Test dough— if it holds together when you pinch it, it doesn't need any more water. If it doesn't come together, add 3 more tablespoons cold water.

4. Remove dough from the food processor, put into a plastic bag, and form into a flat disc. Refrigerate for 30 minutes.

5. Preheat the oven to 400°F. Flour a rolling pin and your counter.

6. Roll out dough to 1/4 inch thickness. Fit dough into an 8- or 9-inch tart pan. Using a fork, slightly puncture bottom of piecrust. Bake for 15 minutes. Remove from the oven, and set aside.

7. In a large skillet over medium heat, add extra-virgin olive oil, yellow onion, garlic, and asparagus, and sauté for 5 minutes.

8. Add spinach, and cook for 3 or 4 more minutes. Remove from heat, and set aside.

9. In a large bowl, whisk together eggs, heavy cream, and ricotta cheese. Add remaining 11/2 teaspoons salt,

Parmesan cheese, paprika, cayenne, black pepper, basil, parsley, and sun-dried tomatoes, and stir to combine.
10. Pour filling into piecrust, and bake for 40 minutes. Remove from the oven, and let rest for 20 minutes before serving warm.

Ricotta Tartine And Honey-roasted Cherry

Servings: 4
Cooking Time: 15 Minutes

Ingredients:
- 4 slices (1/2 inch thick) artisan bread, whole-grain
- 2 cups fresh cherries, pitted
- 2 teaspoons extra-virgin olive oil
- 1/4 cup slivered almonds, toasted
- 1 teaspoon lemon zest
- 1 teaspoon fresh thyme
- 1 tablespoon lemon juice
- 1 tablespoon honey, plus more for serving
- 1 cup ricotta cheese, part-skim
- Pinch of flaky sea salt, such as Maldon
- Pinch of salt

Directions:
1. Preheat oven to 400F. Line a rimmed baking sheet with parchment paper; set aside.
2. In a mixing bowl, toss the cherries with the honey, oil, lemon juice, and salt. Transfer into pan. Roast for about 15 minutes, shaking the pan once or twice during roasting, until the cherries are very soft and warm.

3. Toast the bread. Top with the cheese, the cherries, thyme, lemon zest, almonds, and season with sea salt. If desired, drizzle more honey.

Nutrition Info:Per Serving:320 Cal, 13 g total fat (6 g sat. fat, 6 g mono), 19 mg chol., 272 mg sodium, 401 g pot., 39 g carb.,6 g fiber,2 g sugar, 15 g protein.

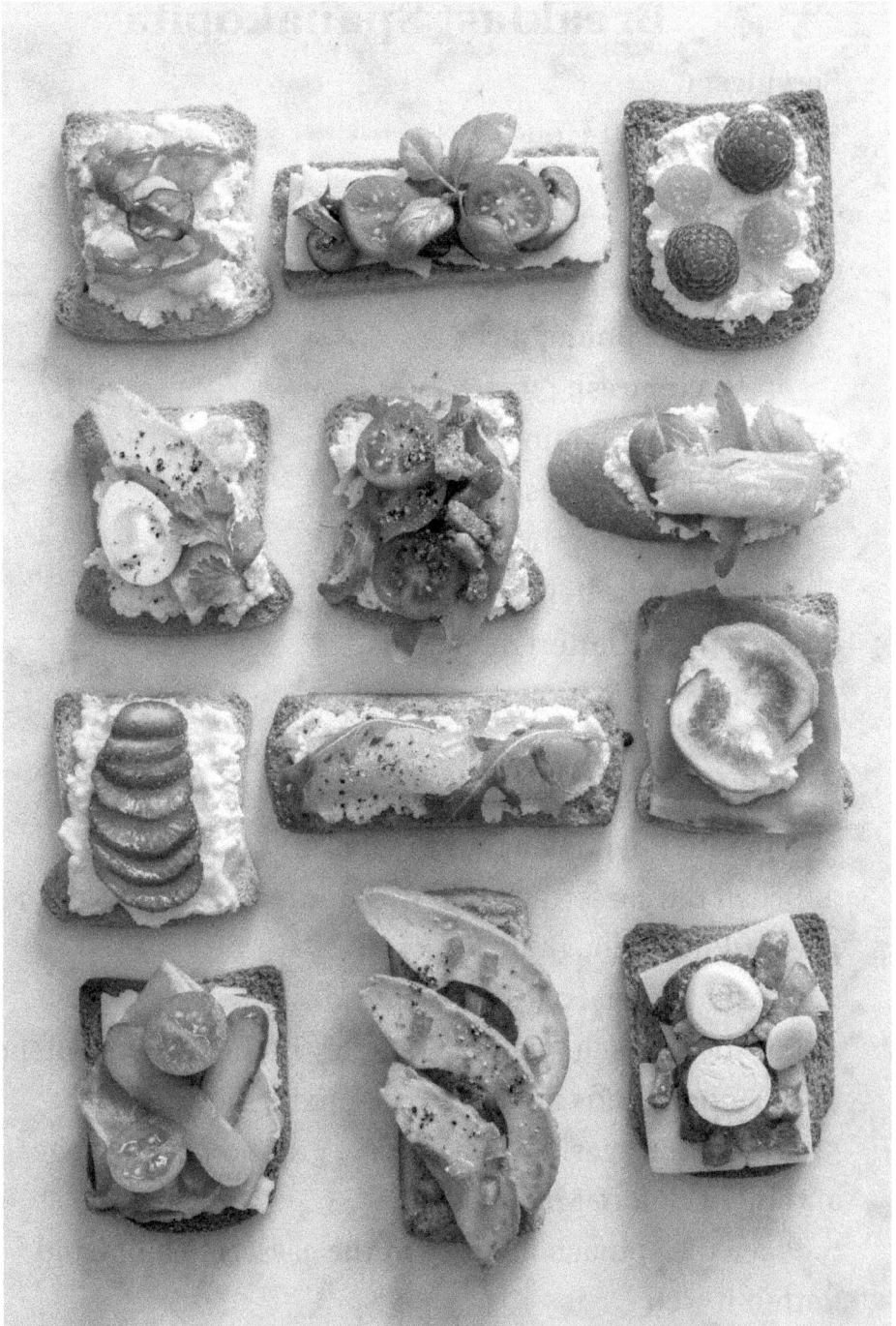

Breakfast Spanakopita

Servings: 6

Cooking Time: 1 Hour

Ingredients:

- 2 cups spinach
- 1 white onion, diced
- ½ cup fresh parsley
- 1 teaspoon minced garlic
- 3 oz Feta cheese, crumbled
- 1 teaspoon ground paprika
- 2 eggs, beaten
- 1/3 cup butter, melted
- 2 oz Phyllo dough

Directions:

1. Separate Phyllo dough into 2 parts.

2. Brush the casserole mold with butter well and place 1 part of Phyllo dough inside.

3. Brush its surface with butter too.

4. Put the spinach and fresh parsley in the blender. Blend it until smooth and transfer in the mixing bowl.

5. Add minced garlic, Feta cheese, ground paprika, eggs, and diced onion. Mix up well.

6. Place the spinach mixture in the casserole mold and flatten it well.

7. Cover the spinach mixture with remaining Phyllo dough and pour remaining butter over it.

8. Bake spanakopita for 1 hour at 350F.

9. Cut it into the servings.

Nutrition Info: Calories 190, fat 15.4, fiber 1.1, carbs 8.4, protein 5.4

Creamy Parsley Soufflé

Servings: 2

Cooking Time: 25 Minutes

Ingredients:

- 2 fresh red chili peppers, chopped
- Salt, to taste
- 4 eggs
- 4 tablespoons light cream
- 2 tablespoons fresh parsley, chopped

Directions:

1. Preheat the oven to 375 degrees F and grease 2 soufflé dishes.

2. Combine all the ingredients in a bowl and mix well.

3. Put the mixture into prepared soufflé dishes and transfer in the oven.

4. Cook for about 6 minutes and dish out to serve immediately.

5. For meal prepping, you can refrigerate this creamy parsley soufflé in the ramekins covered in a foil for about 2-3 days.

Nutrition Info: Calories: 108 Fat: 9g Carbohydrates: 1.1g Protein: 6g Sugar: 0.5g Sodium: 146mg

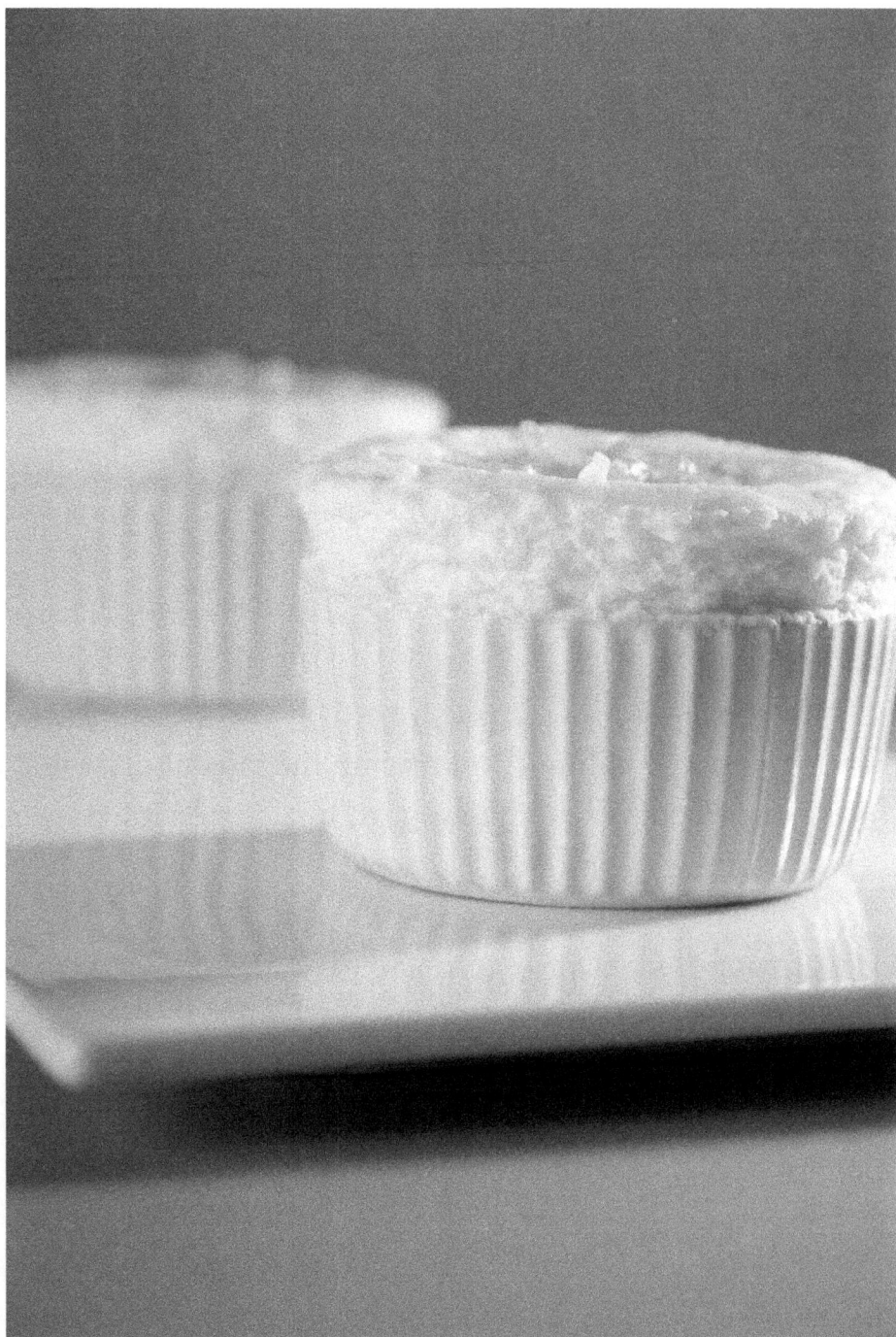

Berry Oats

Servings: 2

Cooking Time: 0 Minutes

Ingredients:
- ½ cup rolled oats
- 1 cup almond milk
- ¼ cup chia seeds
- A pinch of cinnamon powder
- 2 teaspoons honey
- 1 cup berries, pureed
- 1 tablespoon yogurt

Directions:

1. In a bowl, combine the oats with the milk and the rest of the ingredients except the yogurt, toss, divide into bowls, top with the yogurt and serve cold for breakfast.

Nutrition Info: calories 420, fat 30.3, fiber 7.2, carbs 35.3, protein 6.4

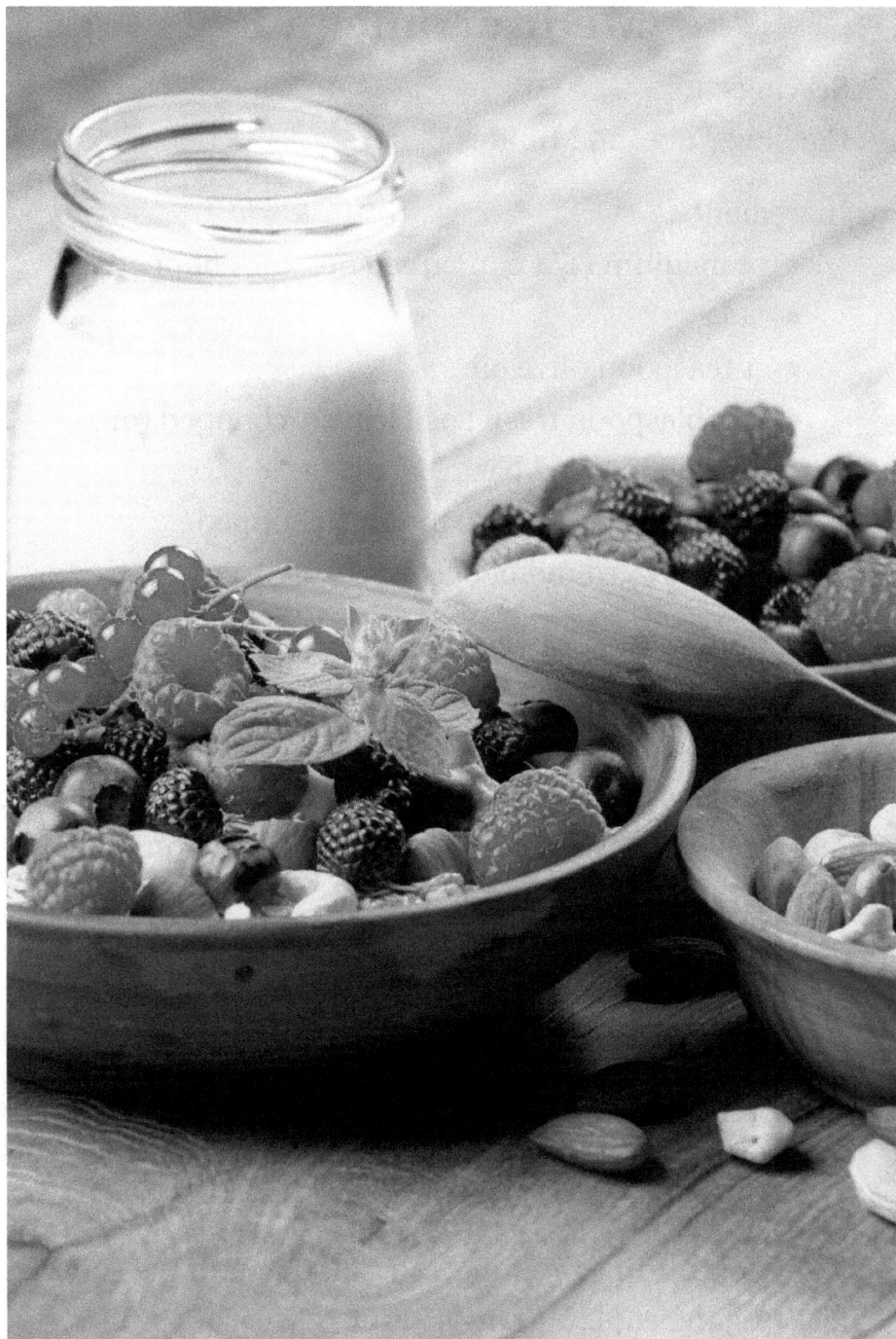

Mediterranean Eggs

Servings: 2

Cooking Time: 15 Minutes

Ingredients:

- 4 medium (1/4 cup) green onions, chopped
- 4 eggs
- 1 teaspoon olive oil
- 1 tablespoon fresh basil leaves, chopped (or 1 teaspoon dried basil leaves)
- 1 medium (3/4 cup) tomato, chopped
- Freshly ground pepper

Directions:

1. In an 8-inch non-stick skillet, heat the olive oil over medium heat. Add onions; cook for about 2 minutes, occasionally stirring. Stir in the tomato and the basil; cook for 1 minute, occasionally stirring, until the tomato is heated through.

2. In a bowl, whisk the eggs; pour over the mixture in the skillet.

3. As the egg mix starts to set, lift with a spatula to allow the uncooked egg to flow underneath; cook for about 3-4 minutes, or until the eggs are thick but still moist. Sprinkle with pepper.

Nutrition Info:Per Serving:190 Cal, 13 g total fat (3.5 g sat. fat), 425 mg chol., 130 mg sodium, 5 g carb.,1 g fiber,3 g sugar, 13 g protein.

Avocado Chickpea Pizza

Servings: 2
Cooking Time: 20 Minutes

Ingredients:
- 1 and ¼ cups chickpea flour
- A pinch of salt and black pepper
- 1 and ¼ cups water
- 2 tablespoons olive oil
- 1 teaspoon onion powder
- 1 teaspoon garlic, minced
- 1 tomato, sliced
- 1 avocado, peeled, pitted and sliced
- 2 ounces gouda, sliced
- ¼ cup tomato sauce
- 2 tablespoons green onions, chopped

Directions:
1. In a bowl, mix the chickpea flour with salt, pepper, water, the oil, onion powder and the garlic, stir well until you obtain a dough, knead a bit, put in a bowl, cover and leave aside for 20 minutes.
2. Transfer the dough to a working surface, shape a bit circle, transfer it to a baking sheet lined with parchment paper and bake at 425 degrees F for 10 minutes.

3. Spread the tomato sauce over the pizza, also spread the rest of the ingredients and bake at 400 degrees F for 10 minutes more.

4. Cut and serve for breakfast.

Nutrition Info: calories 416, fat 24.5, fiber 9.6, carbs 36.6, protein 15.4

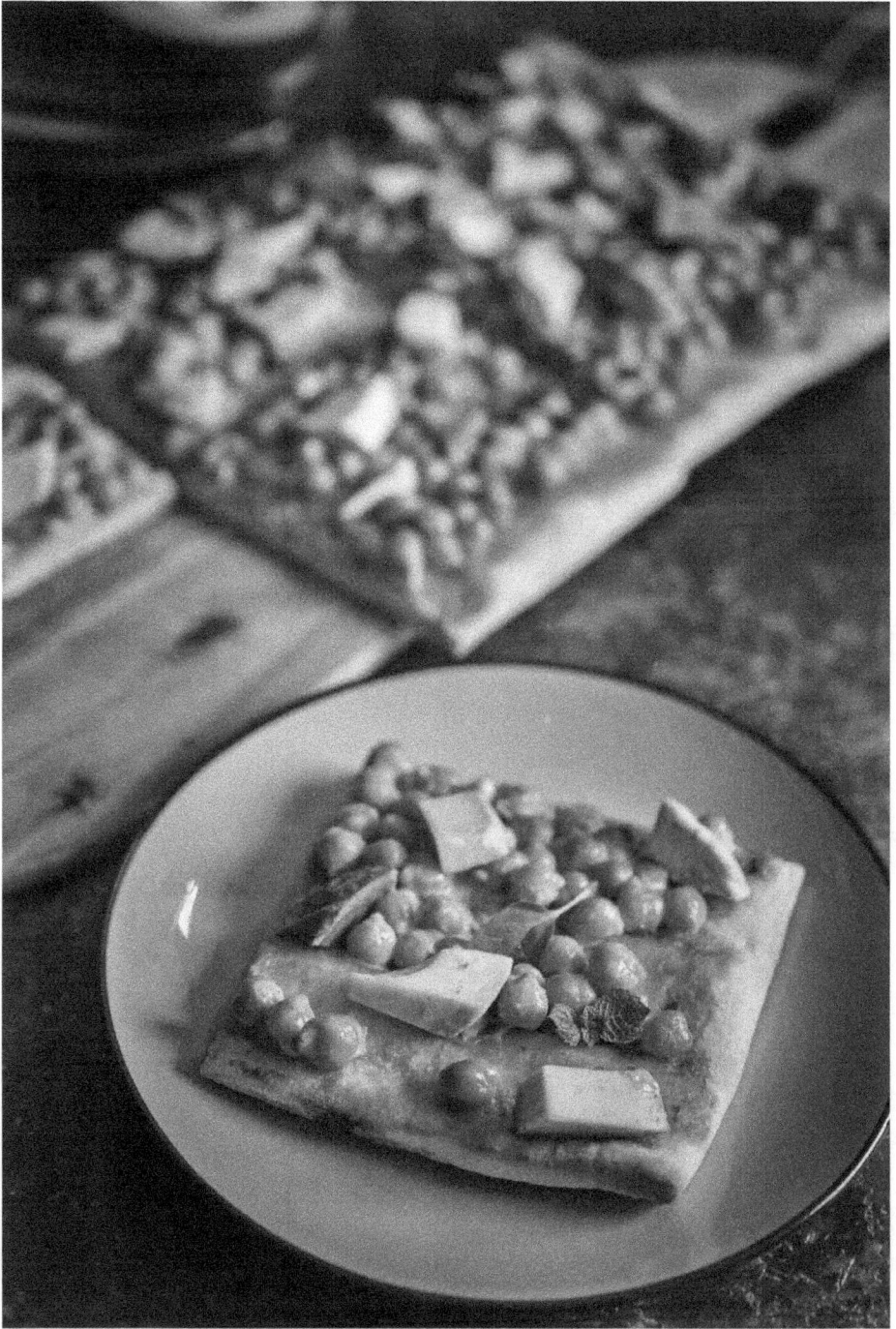

Notes

www.ingramcontent.com/pod-product-compliance
Lightning Source LLC
Chambersburg PA
CBHW050757030426
42336CB00012B/1857